Was that The Sensuous Couple's Guide to Oral Sex

GIVE THE GIFT

Was that an earthquake or did it really feel that good? There is nothing as divine as receiving splendidly performed oral sex. For the woman who wants to give her man the best fellatio ever, and for the man who wants to drive his woman wild with his cunnilingus technique, *The Sensuous Couple's Guide* provides you with the techniques, confidence and skills you need.

Not only will you become a master in the art of oral sex, you will learn how to have fun and enjoy bestowing this remarkable gift on the one you treasure. In clear, concise language, and with a remarkable depth of detail, the authors clearly explain the magic of oral sex in what is, without a doubt, the most complete book on fellatio and cunnilingus available.

TWO BOOKS IN ONE
FLIP OVER FELLATIO

Oral sex is an important part of lovemaking, sometimes considered more special to a man than intercourse. It seems simple enough, but there are methods and practices that can give a man unimaginable pleasure. *The Sensuous Couple's Guide* shows you how to WOW him and enjoy yourself in the process. Guys, this section is for you, too. Help her become an expert in the exciting art of fellatio and you both will go beyond pleasure to ultimate bliss!

Inside you'll discover:

➢ Step by step instructions for giving your man a mind-blowing blowjob.
➢ The anatomy of male sexual arousal - how it works and why.
➢ Effective communication with your partner (his and hers).
➢ Simple – to - advanced techniques.
➢ How to perform (and receive) safe oral sex.
➢ How to introduce oral sex into a new or an established relationship.
➢ How to handle premature, or the lack of, ejaculation, and what to do once it happens.
➢ Advanced "sweet-spot," anal and prostate stimulation for dynamic orgasmic combinations.
➢ How to deal with his or her "issues" and feel comfortable with oral sex.

From setting the scene, convincing your lover (if necessary), through build-up and technique, to a sublime orgasm, Avery Sinclair clearly explains what men want and need. Ladies, give your man everything he wants while simultaneously satisfying your own passions. With *The Sensuous Couple's Guide*, you'll both FLIP OVER fellatio.

Relationships/Sex Instruction

Was that an earthquake?
The Sensuous Couple's Guide to Seismic Oral Sex

GIVE THE GIFT

Was that an earthquake or did it really feel that good? There is nothing as divine as receiving splendidly performed oral sex. For the woman who wants to give her man the best fellatio ever, and for the man who wants to drive his woman wild with his cunnilingus technique, *The Sensuous Couple's Guide* provides you with the techniques, confidence and skills you need.

BUT, not only will you become a master in the art of oral sex, you will learn how to have fun and enjoy bestowing this remarkable gift on the one you treasure. In clear, concise language, and with a remarkable depth of detail, the authors clearly explain the magic of oral sex in what is, without a doubt, the most complete book on fellatio and cunnilingus available.

TWO BOOKS IN ONE
FLIP OVER CUNNILINGUS

Oral sex is an important part of lovemaking, especially for women. From setting the scene, convincing your lover (if necessary), through build-up and technique to a dynamic orgasm, *The Sensuous Couple's Guide* passionately explains exactly what women want. Ladies, this section is for you too. Join together for an exciting adventure in oral sex-beyond pleasure to ultimate bliss!!

Inside you'll learn:

- Step by step instructions for going down on a woman.
- Female anatomy of arousal and what stimulates her most.
- How to perform (and receive) safe oral sex.
- How to introduce oral sex into a new or an established relationship.
- How to handle the disappearing orgasm.
- Advanced G-spot, anal and clitoral stimulation for a dynamic orgasmic combination.
- Proper oral sex etiquette (yes, there is one).
- How to deal with the emotional needs of women.

Rising far above the rest, *The Sensuous Couple's Guide* is male or female specific in the best presented combination of oral sex books ever. With *The Sensuous Couple's Guide*, you'll both FLIP OVER cunnilingus.

Was that an earthquake?

The Sensuous Couple's Guide to Seismic Oral Sex

D. Claire Hutchins
Avery Sinclair

JPS Publishing Company
Dallas, Texas

Was that an earthquake?
The Sensuous Couple's Guide to Seismic Oral Sex
By
D. Claire Hutchins
Avery Sinclair

Published by: JPS Publishing Company, Dallas, Texas
www.jpspublishing.com

All rights reserved. No part of this book may be reproduced or transmitted in any form or by any means, electronic or mechanical, including photocopying, recording or by any information storage and retrieval system without written permission from the publisher, except for the inclusion of brief quotations in a review.

Copyright © 2008 by D. Claire Hutchins and Avery Sinclair

Publisher's Cataloging-in-Publication
(Provided by Quality Books, Inc.)

Hutchins, D. Claire.
  Was that an earthquake? : the sensuous couple's guide to seismic oral sex / D. Claire Hutchins, Avery Sinclair.
  p. cm.
  Includes bibliographical references and index.
  LCCN 2008923254
  ISBN-13: 978-0-9664924-5-3
  ISBN-10: 0-9664924-5-5

  1. Oral sex. 2. Sex instruction. I. Sinclair, Avery. II. Title. III. Title: Sensuous couple's guide to seismic oral sex.

HQ31.5.O73H88 2008   613.9'6
            QBI08-600091

Book One

Cunnilingus

D. Claire Hutchins

Disclaimer

This book provides information regarding the covered subject matter. Neither the publisher nor the authors is engaged in rendering legal, medical, accounting, psychiatric or psychological, or other professional advice. If expert assistance is needed, the services of a professional should be sought.

This book does not contain all the information that is available on this subject. For more information, see the references in the Bibliography section.

The sole purpose of this book is to entertain. The authors and the publisher have no liability or responsibility to any person or entity with respect to any loss or damage caused, or alleged to be caused, directly or indirectly, by the information in this book.

Table of Contents

Book One: Cunnilingus

INDEX TO ILLUSTRATIONS

1   IS THERE ANYTHING BETTER? 1

Why Oral Sex? 1
The History of Cunnilingus 2
Why Do Women Want It? 3
A Man's Point of View 4

2   WHY AND WHERE IT FEELS GOOD: THE ANATOMY OF SEXUAL AROUSAL 6

Anatomy of a Woman 6
A Brief History of Orgasm 11

3   EARTHQUAKE STATUS-THE BEGINNING 15

Getting Started 15
Setting the Mood 25
Setting the Scene 27

4   HOW TO GO DOWN ON A WOMAN 31

The Art of Performing Oral Sex 31
The Clitoris: Step- by- Step 32
Touching Her Emotions 34

5   EARTHQUAKE STATUS FOR THE DETAIL ORIENTED 35

Mouth, Tongue and Hands 35
The Etiquette of Receiving Oral Sex 39
The Worst Mistakes 40

6   VARIATIONS 42

7   THE BALANCE OF POWER: WHO GIVES AND WHO GETS (AND WHY NOT?)! 48

Reciprocation and Fair Play 48

8 THE TOUGH PART: UNDERSTANDING YOUR FEMALE PARTNER 51

A Man's Point of View 51
A Woman's Point of View 52
Combating Sexual Fears 53

9 MORE FUN: VARYING YOUR POSITIONS 55

Cunnilingus Positions 55
Variations 58
Positions for the Disabled or Injured 59

10 DON'T STOP THERE: TAKING IT TO THE NEXT LEVEL 60

G-Spot Stimulation 60
Squirting 61
Ejaculating 62
Anilingus 64

11 DOUBLE DARE: FANTASIES AND BONDAGE 71

Fantasizing 71
Bondage, Sadism and Masochism 75
Safety Tips 76
Sex Toys 77
Tongue Piercing 79
Curious Facts about Oral Sex 79

12 ADVANCED INTIMACY: SOME THINGS YOU MIGHT NOT WANT TO THINK ABOUT 80

Menstruation 81
Pregnancy 82
Medical Problems That Affect Sexuality 83
Non-orgasmic 83
PC Muscles 84
Maintaining an Erection 85
Pain and Cramping 86
Exercises 86
Blowing into the Vagina 87
Oral Sex after Ejaculation 87

13	**THE UNFUN PART: SAFE SEX AND SEXUALLY TRANSMITTED DISEASES**	**88**

Women's Sexuality..*88*
AIDS..*90*
Bacterial STDs..*91*
Other STDs...*92*
Protection...*94*
Monogamy..*96*
Protecting Yourself..*96*
Teenagers and Oral Sex.....................................*97*

14	**QUESTIONS AND ANSWERS**	**102**

Aversion to Oral Sex..*102*
Does Diet Affect Taste?....................................*104*
Helping Him Improve.......................................*104*
Asking for Oral Sex..*105*
Kissing After Oral Sex.....................................*106*
Sixty-Nine..*107*
Vaginal Farts...*107*

15	**GIVING CAN BE AS GOOD AS GETTING**	**109**
16	**THE EMOTIONAL NEEDS OF WOMEN**	**113**

Early History...*113*
Why Women Love...*114*

INDEX **117**

BIBLIOGRAPHY & GLOSSARY **121**

Illustrations credits

Original artwork by Sed Kaya, Sed Kaya Productions, Winter Garden, Florida

Historical and other drawings in Public Domain

Cover by Juanita Dix, Florida

The Authors

Avery Sinclair and D. Claire Hutchins are teachers and sex educators who reside in the suburbs of Dallas, Texas.

Illustrations - Cunnilingus

Figure 1: Drawing by Édouard-Henri Avril .... Frontpiece
Figure 2: Terrace Reliefs of Kha-juraho's Laksman Temple d. 954 3
Figure 3: Watercolor by Achille Devéria (1800-1857) 4
Figure 4: External Genitalia 7
Figure 5: Human Vulva 10
Figure 6: Bathe or Shower Together 25
Figure 7: Massage 28
Figure 8: Cunnilingus 33
Figure 9: The 69 Position 44
Figure 10: The 68 Position 45
Figure 11: Classic Cunnilingus Position 56
Figure 12: Face Sitting 57
Figure 13: Anilingus 69
Figure 14: Light Bondage and Role Playing 75
Figure 15: Dildo 77
Figure 16: Simple Plastic Vibrator 78
Figure 17: Pregnancy 82
Figure 18: True Intimacy Means Safety 95
Figure 19: Enjoying Each Other 112

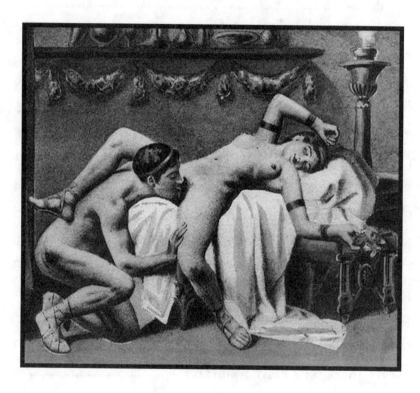

Figure 1: Drawing by Édouard-Henri Avril

1843-1928

1 Is There Anything Better?

Why Oral Sex?

Ahhhh! Nothing feels like oral sex, and most couples will try it at one time or another. Men admit that they enjoy giving oral sex and women certainly enjoy receiving it. Few tools can equal the tongue for the amount of pleasure it delivers. Women love it—it is the height of pure sexual pleasure.

The intimacy and sexual closeness that cunnilingus provides is highly arousing and can add a potent sexual spark between couples who practice it. Like a new sex toy, adding oral sex to your sexual routine can open up exciting channels of intimacy.

For men, cunnilingus is a powerful lovemaking technique that has no relationship to the size of his penis. In this respect, at least, all men are created equal. (Unless you are Gene Simmons, who is definitely not equal.) Giving the intimacy of oral sex shows your partner that you love her and want her to be sexually fulfilled. Orgasm, affection, intimacy and having fun should be the main goals.

Cunnilingus is used in both homosexual and

heterosexual relationships. In a heterosexual relationship, it can also be a method of contraception. For those women dedicated to virginity, it is not considered sex (not exactly, anyway), and it does not involve a loss of virginity.

The History of Cunnilingus

Cunnilingus is by no means a modern invention. It is an age-old practice that can be traced back to illustrations of oral sex on pottery as early as 300 BC all the way to modern times. Scrolls from China and Japan dated 200 BC contain cunnilingus drawings. The Kama Sutra, written in 400 AD, includes oral sex. Ancient erotic art has many referrals to oral sex such as the explicit "yoni kisses" in 12th century Indian temple carvings (*see Figure 2*).

In ancient Rome, before the Christians, sexual acts were viewed as acts of submission or control. For example, it was disgusting for a male to perform fellatio or cunnilingus, since that would mean he was penetrated. It was considered acceptable to receive fellatio from a woman, however. Equally acceptable was oral sex from a man of lower social status, such as a slave or debtor.

Oral sex was also considered more shameful than anal sex. Those who practiced oral sex were supposed to have foul breath and were unwelcome at a dinner table. It was taboo for public health reasons also because genitals were considered unclean.

Cunnilingus has a special place in Chinese Taoism. The aim of Taoism is to achieve immortality, or at least longevity, and the loss of semen, vaginal, and other bodily liquids is believed to bring about a corresponding loss of vitality. Conversely, by either semen retention or ingesting the secretions from the vagina, a male or female can conserve and increase his/her *ch'i,* or original vital breath.

Cunnilingus

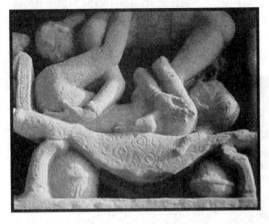

Figure 2: Terrace Reliefs of Kha-juraho's Laksman Temple d. 954

Today, many cultures and parts of the world, not to mention religions, frown upon cunnilingus. Some of the reasons are that it does not lead to procreation; it may also be considered a humiliating or an unclean practice.

The Names of Cunnilingus

Cunnilingus is sometimes referred to as "gelling the hair," "drinking from the red river," "dining at the Y (DATY)," "licking out," "picking the daisies," "licking the peach," "going down" or "eating out," "smack clam," "munch rug," "dining at the pink taco stand," "muff-diving," "carpet-munching," "feasting," "harvesting the salmon" and "eating the flower". In lesbian culture several common slang terms used are "giving lip," "lip service," or "tipping the velvet."

Why Do Women Want It?

An orgasm from cunnilingus is fast, relaxing and healing. Done right, it can bring a woman to heights of pleasure she has never experienced before. She will feel appreciated, respected, desired and admired.

Many women complain that they don't get oral sex as often as they want, and when they do, their partner often doesn't do it right **Guys, remember this: men who perform great oral sex are always in demand.**

Compared to penetrative sex, oral sex done right has a greater chance of bringing your partner to orgasm. Many women prefer it to intercourse because they find that, other than masturbation, it is the easiest way to achieve orgasm. There are some women who refuse to date a man who doesn't or won't go down on them. By the first date, they are able to weed out those who won't perform oral sex and refuse to go out with them again. If it's important to her (and it is to most women), and if the man says no to oral sex, a woman can stop the relationship before it gets too serious. That way, she won't have to spend the rest of her life giving, but never receiving, oral sex. I would highly recommend that you do the same. A man who finds a woman's genitals distasteful is not the kind of man you want to be hooked up with for life (or even five minutes).

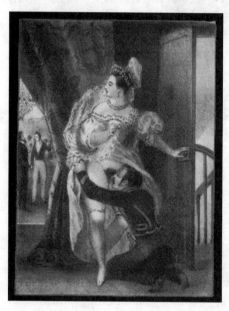

Figure 3: Watercolor by Achille Devéria (1800-1857)

Women love oral sex for the same reason men love oral sex—to be truly loved. When they receive cunnilingus, women don't feel used or abused as if they were housemaids or cooks. It elevates them above being just a friend. It makes them true partners, perhaps for life. Oral sex proves to a woman that she is fully accepted as a sexual being. Every part of her is loved and accepted by her lover and partner.

A Man's Point of View

Do men enjoy giving oral sex? Most men perform oral

Cunnilingus

sex to give the woman pleasure. Often, they find that participating in this delight arouses them as well.

Cunnilingus is a fundamental part of the whole lovemaking experience. It is the perfect time for a man to learn what his partner likes and what she needs to become fully aroused. Without oral sex, this information may be difficult to come by. For some men, the smell, taste and closeness of cunnilingus are their biggest turn-ons. Others enjoy being "used" as "sex toys." There is nothing to compare to the sexual intimacy and enhanced lovemaking provided by oral sex.

Why would a man deny himself the ecstasy of orally pleasuring his woman? Even though most women love receiving oral sex, there are some men who do not love giving it. There are many reasons, but one of the primary ones is that going down on a woman isn't exactly easy. It is one of the most difficult sexual acts to perform successfully. It takes refined skill combined with patience, healthy free-flowing communication and lots of energy for the long haul. But hang in there. We created this book to enlighten you. We will help make oral sex—one of the most beautiful and intimate activities in the world—an easy and enjoyable part of your lovemaking routine.

Guys, you can learn to enjoy giving cunnilingus almost as much as she likes getting it!

2
Why and Where It Feels Good: The Anatomy of Sexual Arousal

Most of us are so hung up about our bodies that we are too ashamed to study each other's body parts. If a man wants to perform fantastic oral sex, it is extremely helpful for him to know as much as possible about the female body. Not knowing is worse than being ineffective. It's too easy to end up fumbling and embarrassed.

Unfortunately, the erotic parts of the female body do not automatically draw fingers, tongues and penises in the right direction. Fumbling around in the dark doesn't help much, especially since the anatomy of each woman varies so much. Anyone who makes love to a woman should take the time and trouble to admire what she's got between her legs and learn all about her physical parts.

Anatomy of a Woman

Each woman's genitals are unique, differing in

Cunnilingus

appearance, size, shape and color. Even though they are unique, their appearance has nothing to do with her response to stimulation.

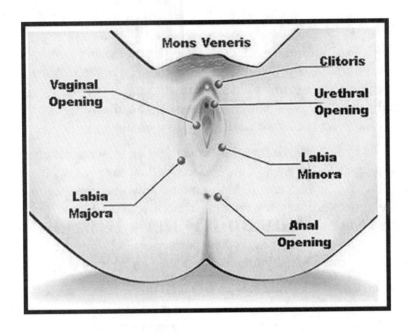

Figure 4: External Genitalia

External Anatomy

Look directly at a naked woman. The visible area, the area over the pubic bone, is the pubic mound. It is named after the goddess of love, Venus—mons veneris, which means the mound of Venus. This area is usually covered with hair, although these days it can be bikini groomed or even shaved completely. The mons tapers down between her thighs and splits like a cleft around the vaginal opening. If the woman then sits with her legs apart, viz-a-viz, Sharon Stone in Basic Instinct, one can see the outer lips of the vagina, the labia. The labia have soft folds that are different in each woman. They are usually the same color as the other skin of her body and are usually covered with hair. Some have dark, thick pubic hair and others have fine, wispy hair. Some women may shave. The bare flesh ranges in color from pale pink to dark brown. It may be two-toned. This area is comparable to the male scrotum and is formed from the same tissue while a baby is *in utero*.

The Clitoris

Positioning. Nestled between the protruding labia is the tip of the clitoris or "glans." The slightly bulb shaped head of the clitoral shaft is not a gland. In this instance, "glans" means a small round mass or body and tissue that can swell or harden. This is a pretty accurate description of what the clitoris does.

Pre-1960s. Before the 1960s, few knew what the clitoris was, much less what to call it. That's when the word "clitoris" came into common usage. Many men and women were ignorant of its function. Early sex manuals described it as a "mini-penis." This completely incorrect analogy led to numerous problems when men, trying to please their partners, would rub the clitoris with the same intensity they wanted used on their penises.

Female Genitalia. In females, the external sex organs are collectively called the vulva. The parts making up the vulva include the mons pubis, labia majora and minora, clitoris, and greater vestibular glands.

Iceberg Tip. Although the word "clitoris" is often used as a catch-all term that refers to all of a woman's sex organs, this is actually only partly true. The entire female genitalia does not consist of separate and distinct parts. The area underneath the inner and outer lips (labia), the ring around the urethra (where it leaves the body) and the wall of the perineum all contain erectile tissues that fill with blood and swell upon arousal.

Although the clitoris used to be considered the small part that protrudes between the labia, that is actually merely the tip of the clitoris. We now know that the whole area is interconnected with an intricate web of muscles, nerves and blood vessels. All react and engage with one another when aroused. The clitoris is actually much bigger than we supposed, and it is far larger than what is described in most sex guides and anatomy texts. The little nub of hard flesh is the tip of the iceberg.

Beginning at the top of a wishbone shape which houses the clit, two sides fork down around the vagina. The entire glans, the internal clitoris, begins at one end of the shaft of the vagina and continues into the surrounding hard tissue. Its wings (technically crura) extend into the walls of the vagina. The area occupied by the clitoris and crura is actually a complex clitoral system.

Several layers of muscles line the pelvic floor, connecting the clit to the erectile tissues. An oval shaped muscle of erectile tissue surrounds the inner lips and clit where the vagina and urethra pass through it. It connects to another oval that surrounds the anal sphincter muscle and encircles the anus.

The crura are surrounded by spongy erectile tissue in a pair of corpora cavernosa with a similar structure to the male. During arousal, nitric oxide is released to effect relaxation of the cavernosal artery and nearby muscle in a process that is similar to male arousal. More blood flows in through the clitoral cavernosal artery, the pressure in the clitoris rises, and the clitoris becomes hard and engorged with blood. This leads to expulsion of the glans clitoris and enhanced sensitivity to physical contact. The crua clitoris is simply a continuation of the clitoris on either side of the corpus cavernosa. The two greater vestibular bulbs or glands expand at the same time as the glans clitoris. Blood flow to the genitals increases and squeezes the inner sides of the vagina. All of the woman's erectile tissue will swell.

Hood. The wealth of sensual tissue in the female vagina is no excuse to ignore the main attraction. The outer clitoris is still the most active and sensitive part of the female sex organ. It needs all the attention a man (or woman) can give it. Its protective covering, called the "hood," is analogous to a man's foreskin. It protects the clit and diffuses the sensations of touch. Some women find having the clitoral hood touched too intense and prefer indirect stimulation through the vulva.

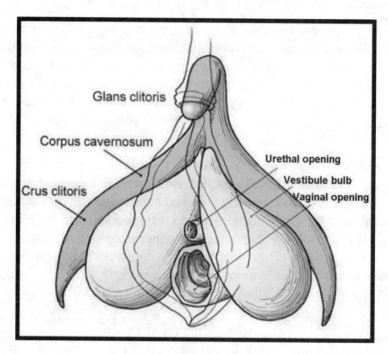

Figure 5: Human Vulva

Sometimes all it takes to expose the tip is to pull back the hood. Sometimes it doesn't become visible until the woman is aroused. At first, it is usually too sensitive to stimulate directly. In the early stages of arousal, it may be actually painful. **So begin with indirect stimulation.** Kiss and nibble her entire body, avoiding the genital area. Get her used to your touch while you get used to the aroma and taste of her skin. Take time to discover the parts where she gets the most stimulation. The best approach to a woman's genitals is anything but direct.

The clitoris is richly endowed with 8000 nerve endings. It contains more nerve endings than any other part of a human body, whether male or female—more than the fingertips,

Cunnilingus

tongue, anus, and twice as many as the entire penis. The clitoris has only one job—to give pleasure. For most women, stimulation of the clitoris is essential to orgasm.

Before you touch the clitoris, make sure the clitoris is wet. It does not have any moisture of its own and is extremely sensitive. As we have cautioned previously, be sure to work up to touching the clit. It is far too delicate to be handled until the woman is aroused.

A Brief History of Orgasm

Pre-1970s

Three Types of Sexual Experience. For young people in the late 1960s and early 1970s, there were three types of sexual experience. One, you could get yourself off by hand. This was the most common sexual experience since it required no social skill or effort, and anybody could do it. If you were lucky enough to have a boyfriend or girlfriend, your eyes met, your hands and lips touched, you talked on the phone and were happy to be alive and in love. Occasionally, having a boyfriend or girlfriend meant that you progressed to intercourse or, as it was known then, "going all the way." Sex before marriage was slowly starting to become acceptable.

1970s

Change of Life. In the 1970s, life, and especially sex, changed dramatically. With the introduction of the birth control pill, sex before marriage became more widely acceptable.

It is impossible to underestimate the impact of the pill on the American way of life. It granted more freedom to do what came naturally. Gone were some of the old inhibitions, especially since having unwanted children was no longer a problem. Other factors that helped change the sexual climate included the invasion of rock'n'roll bands from Britain, the use of LSD and other psychedelic drugs, the media, marijuana, the mini-skirt, the women's movement and the antiwar movement.

Intercourse Insufficient. Sex was a wide open

experience, but was that the best of all possible worlds? Not necessarily. Most men didn't know a lot about what a woman needed, and often intercourse was way too fast. Partners were too inexperienced. Women started to ask themselves if they were getting the most out of their sexual experiences. When the answer was a resounding "NO," female orgasm was a subject that began to be discussed.

Those of us alive during this time were conditioned by society to believe that intercourse was the only "real" way to have sex. However, with "real sex," women weren't always enjoying the experience as much as their male partners. Since many women find it impossible to orgasm when vaginal penetration is the only form of stimulation, intercourse left them feeling incomplete and unfinished. With the sexual revolution, women became freer to explore new ways to express their sexuality. They soon learned that there were many ways to "get off."

Once they could enjoy orgasms other than with penetrative sex, that didn't make their orgasms any less "real."

Vaginal vs. Clitoral Orgasm. A theory, originally propounded by Sigmund Freud, stated that clitoral orgasms were "immature" and that only orgasm achieved through vaginal intercourse was "mature." This was based in part on the idea that masturbation was an immature practice. Therefore, orgasms coming from direct stimulation of the clitoris were also immature.

Modern Times

It was up to Masters and Johnson to publish findings on female sexuality that demolished Freud's idea of mature vaginal orgasms. Masters and Johnson found that all orgasms center on the clitoris and classifying orgasm as vaginal or clitoral was incorrect. Now that we know the clitoris encompasses a much larger area than previously supposed, descending into the vaginal canal itself, that finding makes more sense. The strict separation into vaginal and clitoral orgasms is artificial and misleading.

However, the mistaken classifications of "vaginal" and "clitoral" are still very much alive and hound women with their supposed inability to achieve the ideal orgasm. These views are still widely held and often imposed from a male perspective.

The clitoris and the vagina are not two distinct areas of the female anatomy. Rather than being the centers of erotic sensation, both are parts of the same structure. A woman on the verge of orgasm experiences diffuse sensations that permeate the whole genital area and sometimes the whole body. Therefore, what used to be called a "clitoral" orgasm, sometimes not through intercourse, is no different from a "vaginal" orgasm achieved through intercourse. It has actually stimulated the clitoris as well. There is no such thing as a "wrong" or a "right" orgasm.

Each Woman's Orgasm Is Unique

No two orgasms are exactly alike, and no two women get off in exactly the same way. Some women started at four to have orgasms and some at sixty-four. Some women expect an orgasm every time; and some women are content not to have orgasms at all. They would be happy, that is, if they weren't made to feel abnormal or freakish.

Some women prefer indirect stimulation or orgasms by pressure alone—like pressing the thighs together and tensing the muscles rythmetically. Some women prefer water stimulation and enjoy orgasms in the bathtub with a shower massager or in a whirlpool in front of a jet stream. Orgasms can be mild to intense, alone or with a partner. Some women ejaculate, some enjoy penetration, some have huge orgasms, others have little ones, some have multiple orgasms, and some women have only one. Some women are not particularly sexual, but may become so. Learning to orgasm is like learning to ride a bicycle. After hours of struggle and practice, continually falling off and becoming frustrated, suddenly everything clicks. When it does, the woman is in for a ride she will want to repeat over and over. The more she does so, just as with bike riding, the better at it she will become.

Each woman needs to explore her own unique sexuality. While one woman might love and need oral sex, another might crave a penis in her vagina. Another might crave both. Communication is the key to letting our man know which kind of woman we are.

If it is oral sex that you crave, whether with or without sex, this guide will lead you and your partner through all the feelings, preparations and actions, step-by-step.

3 Earthquake Status-The Beginning

Getting Started

Some women have a problem with oral sex because they are not communicating what they want to their lovers. Or they may be afraid to truly let go in front of another person.

How to Ask for Oral Sex

If you've never had oral sex with a partner, either because they are new or because of some other reason, it is okay to ask for oral sex. Demanding, however, doesn't work—at least not in the long run. Perhaps your partner may have been immovable about giving oral sex in the past. In that case, try hinting that if he pleases you, you'll take care of him. If you've been performing fellatio without reciprocation, you can cut him off. You might even suggest a "69" position. You can work cunnilingus into your regular sexual program, but don't expect it every time. Afterwards, you can reward him by reciprocating with fellatio, indulging him in one of his fantasies or by performing another favorite sex act.

Communication

Through Words. Communicate your desires openly and without shame. If you stumble over the actual words, sometimes it is easier to show than tell. You can demonstrate what feels the best for your lover by showing him what you do when you masturbate. Try placing your lover's hand over yours as you touch yourself. Have him copy what you did to yourself. Most men are going to be thrilled. You are sharing your body with him, and he will love it.

Through Touch. Let your partner examine your body. Open up the labia, gently pulling the lips apart, and let him look. He may even want to lick the inner lips. You can spread the lips (labia) until you find the clit. Sometimes the distance of the clitoris from the vaginal opening varies greatly. Or the clitoris may be completely hooded, which is called an "embedded clitoris."

The clitoris may be difficult to see, but it will be easy to feel, especially after you reach a state of excitement. Just because they come in different sizes and locations doesn't mean a thing for your capacity to orgasm. All clitorises work just fine.

Some women fear that they will take too long to reach orgasm. Men should reassure their partners that pleasure is the goal, not orgasm. That way, she can lie back and enjoy herself.

Sense of Humor

One of the principal problems with oral sex is the lack of playfulness. Partners approach it like they have a difficult job to do. Oral sex is a natural act that flows out of healthy desire. Don't let it become laden with issues. If it becomes something we are afraid of or something we want desperately, then we can become terrified of failing at it. Instead of trying to make it a flawless performance, and this goes for the giver as well as the

Cunnilingus

receiver, approach it with a sense of fun and playfulness. Otherwise, instead of being perfect and romantic, it will end up being filled with tension and awkwardness.

Oral sex is a giddy experiment with another person's body. An investigation that seeks pleasure and a fantastic gift, oral sex can also be thought of as naughty or nasty by some. Don't worry. Being naughty and nasty can make you feel adventurous and wicked when you perform or receive cunnilingus, which can be a great stimulus to orgasm. Others may view it as a sacred act of worship. Be open and receptive to all of your feelings, the sacred and profane, and you will enjoy oral sex to the ultimate.

Taste, Smell and Appearance

Social Shame. Women grow up with a tremendous amount of sexual shame. It has been taught them since they were born. Consequently, having a partner so close to her genitals may be scary and conjure up powerful body image issues. Her fears center on how her body smells, looks or tastes. Women learn early on that their vaginas are dirty, proven by douche and tampon commercials. There is also theological backing for this idea from more than a few religions. Even the most beautiful woman is shy about her body.

Dating from the first centuries AD, the ancient Indian writings describe oral sex, discussing fellatio in great detail. They only briefly mention cunnilingus. According to the *Kama Sutra*, fellatio was mostly practiced by eunuchs, who used their mouths as substitutes for female genitalia. According to these ancient writings, fellatio was also practiced by "unchaste women." The widespread tradition in that country is that cunnilingus is degrading and unclean. The *Kama Sutra* followed suit by asserting that a "wise man" should not engage in that form of intercourse, while acknowledging that it could be appropriate in some unspecified cases.

Men, when you begin to perform the act of oral sex, tact is of the utmost importance. Even though they may enjoy receiving oral sex, women often have trouble getting over the feeling that they are smelly or dirty. Reassure your partner, if need be. Far from degrading or unclean, any kiss is the first taste of her. Her odors, tastes and appearance define her uniqueness. When you first taste her, it will be a satisfying learning experience.

Taste

Women today often wear clothing that prevents adequate circulation of air around the genitals. To prepare for oral sex, a woman needs to rinse her genitals in plain water at the very least. Rinse thoroughly between the folds of the labia and the head and shaft of the clitoris. Flavored lubricants are a possibility. They come in every flavor, including peanut butter, pina colada and champagne. Generally, however, you will want to avoid them because they contain sugar which is disastrous to the friendly lactobacilli in your vagina. If you are nervous, however, about how you taste, masturbate and then smell your fingers afterward, or try a taste. This is what your lover will taste. Most lovers will find it a highly arousing aphrodisiac.

The taste of your vulva can range from slightly tangy to slippery saltiness to having a hint of iron if it is around time for the menstrual cycle. You may not have the same sweetness every day of the month, which is normal. A noticeable change might warrant a health check. The many chemicals and pheromones in the female body act as powerful aphrodisiacs. That doesn't guarantee, however, that your body chemistry—smell, taste and feel—will "click" with your chosen lover. Hopefully, it will.

If you are the one giving the cunnilingus, make sure you tell your woman how much you love her taste. This will turn her on even more and help her let go and enjoy the experience. Plus, she will never forget you. One lover told me my vagina had a slightly sweet taste. I have never forgotten him.

A common concern with women is that what they eat affects the smell and taste of their vaginas.

There is no scientific research on the subject—only anecdotal evidence, but it is widely believed that what you ingest can affect the smell and taste of your vaginal secretions. Your taste depends on a number of things. For example, if you've ingested garlic, linguini or multivitamins, any of them may affect the way your genitals taste. However, there's no surefire recipe to guarantee that you'll always taste great. Plus, it depends on how your individual body chemistry reacts with what you eat. It's like perfume. A brand is the same in the bottle, but it reacts differently to the body chemistry of every individual who wears it. It smells differently on different people.

If your boyfriend already enjoys giving you oral sex, he most likely enjoys your special flavor and aroma. But, if you want to play it safe, stick to a diet with lots of vegetables, fruits and whole grains. Try to avoid foods that affect your breath and body smell, such as garlic, asparagus, spices (like curry) and excess amounts of dairy and animal products.

Smell

Smells Like Yogurt. A naturally healthy vagina has a slightly pungent, sweet odor similar to plain yogurt. Plain yogurt at room temperature has practically the same bacteria as a healthy, juicy vagina because the same lactobacilli exist in both environments. These friendly bacteria protect the vagina. The ebb and flow of chemicals and hormones maintain the bacterial balance necessary to sustain a healthy vaginal ecosystem.

PH Balance. On any given day, the skin's pH is between 6.0 and 7.0 while the healthy vagina hovers between 3.8 and 4.5. To compare: black coffee is pH5; lemon is pH2; wine has the same pH as the vagina. The lactic acid in vaginal secretions plays a big role in keeping the pH low.

Delicate pH may be knocked askew when undesirable bacteria outnumber the friendly lactobacilli. Secretions may take on a stronger smell. It doesn't take much to upset the system. A too-alkaline mixture produces an unpleasant odor. There can be a number of causes, but douching, soap and semen are the worst offenders. Ejaculate is 8 pH, which is more alkaline than saliva, tears or sweat.

Douching alone is one of biggest causes of vaginal infections. Over-washing with regular soap, not washing thoroughly, or using body soaps that are not pH balanced can upset the system. Pay attention to your body. Your odor tells you to do something about it.

Hygiene. Quit feeling "dirty." The best test for adequate genital hygiene is to insert a finger inside your vagina, make a few circles, and then smell and taste yourself. Once you've decided that's not so awful, do it at different times of the day and different times of the month. Smells tend to alter throughout the monthly cycle. Get to know yourself. Even if you don't like it, that doesn't mean your partner feels the same. If you are in need of attention, then get it.

Wash up before oral sex. A bath or shower before is ideal. Switch to soaps with a lower pH. Natural body soaps tend to have less pH than the typical kind. Avoid lubricants that contain glycerin, a kind of sugar, which leads to yeast infections. You will also want to avoid oils and oily soaps that make the body work overtime to flush them out.

Men, take time to become accustomed to the scent of your lover's skin by gently massaging the vulva with your hand. Try the taste of her on your fingers. At this point, you can change your mind before you perform cunnilingus or go forward confidently to discover the true sweetness of her smell and taste.

Appearance

Many women, sadly, don't feel "normal" down there. Almost every woman is shy about her body and even the most gorgeous woman will worry about how you like her body and her genital area. One woman confided to me that her image of her genitals was an ugly one.

Cunnilingus

> Men have 'gone down' on me, but I was always much too uncomfortable to reach an orgasm. The thought of someone licking my genitals seemed unsanitary. Worse yet, my partner could see everything. I only allowed cunnilingus for a few moments before I pulled my lover back on top of me for 'normal sex.'

Although no two female genital areas are exactly alike, they all have the same equipment. All have hair, outer labia, unmatched inner labia, a clit, and a slit. It is NORMAL to be different. They come in different sizes, colors and shapes; some are tucked inside like a little girl and some have thick luscious lips. Some are nested in bushes of hair and others are covered with transparent fuzz. There are designs, shapes and patterns similar to Mother Nature: shells, flowers, perhaps an orchid. The outer lips can be full and rounded or tight, trim and flat. On some women the inner labia are hidden and nearly flush to surrounding tissue. On others, they can be distinct, even long or fluted, and might rest outside the outer labia. The inner labia come in various lengths and shapes. The clitoris can be substantial and thick or a petite ridge or anywhere in between.

Men learn much of what they know from soft porn, or "split beaver" photographs. "Beaver" is slang for female genitals and "split beaver" is slang for when a woman holds her genitals open. We may feel that it is degrading for these women to expose themselves in garter belts and black net stockings. Regardless, they have vulvas just like ours. We can learn that we are not ugly or deformed from these photographs. Men know it already, obviously.

If you are the giver of cunnilingus, your partner may worry about what you think of her. Naturalness and openness may have to be learned. For your part, admire her body. Appreciate your woman's unique qualities and tell her what makes her special. Because women are more verbal than men, they will respond to your verbal cues, especially during lovemaking. But when they find someone who revels in their taste and smell, there is nothing hotter. When a woman lets go completely, it's a fantastic experience for you both. There's a lot more to oral sex than orgasm. It's about making your lover feel good all over.

Cleanliness

The vagina is the cleanest place in the body, cleaner even than the mouth. Nonetheless, cleaning it is still important. To prepare for oral sex, use a hypoallergenic soap with low pH that you can find at drugstores. Since the mouth is even less hygienic than the vagina, men will want to wash up there too.

Pubic hair

Even though everyone's got it, when it comes to oral sex, pubic hair may be a matter of concern. Some people love the feel, taste and texture, but for others, renegade hairs can be a real turn off. To dislodge any stray hairs, women should run their fingers gently through their public hair before oral sex. Maybe you have a special little comb you can use to get the stray hairs out. Just be sure teeth are wide-set. During oral sex, an option for your partner is to gently hold the outer labia open with his fingers to keep any hair out of the way.

Women may consider lightly trimming the area where the outer lips turn to inner lips and the area above the clitoral hood. This shows off the vulva slightly and most men enjoy it. As an alternative, you can put your partner in charge of the weekly trim and consider it a part of foreplay.

Shaving

Begin by taking a shower or warm bath to soften the pubic hair. Using a small pair of scissors, like mustache trimmers, trim the pubic area. To decrease irritation, rub a bit of oil onto the skin, like almond or olive, being sure not to get the oil inside your vagina. Try using a hair conditioner to further soften the area, then lather well with a shaving cream or gel. Using a disposable razor or an electric trimmer, shave in the

Cunnilingus

same direction that the hair grows. Using as few strokes as possible, rinse the razor in warm water after every pass. Don't dry shave! Using a mirror and sitting on a towel, shave the edges of the outer labia carefully, stretching them out flat with your hand.

When finished, rinse off with a gentle soap, pat dry and apply a scent-free, hypoallergenic lotion. Never use body powders as they contain talc, which has been linked with cervical cancer. You may partially shave the area, leaving a little "landing strip" of hair or you can completely shave the whole area.

Be sure and reshave regularly, avoiding any stubble that will abrade your partners face, lips or tongue. If you haven't shaved recently and are concerned about stubble, you may shield your pubic bone with your hand if you are in the midst of passion and don't want to take the time to shave. This probably should be used only with a partner who is on intimate terms with you: you are trying to protect his face, not hide the stubble.

A hypoallergenic lotion will help any itching as the hair grows back. If you develop an uncomfortable, ugly, red rash of bumps, you have razor burn. Beware of over-the-counter and prescription creams as they contain cortisone, which can cause thinning of the skin. To avoid razor burn, splash the area with cool water after shaving. Use calendula creams or ointments and use a natural aftershave.

The hair around the anus may also be trimmed with a small pair of scissors or it can also be shaved. It can be quite a reach for you. Perhaps your lover can do it as a part of foreplay.

Waxing

For those who want to clean up the genital area even more, you can try waxing. There is a warm wax specifically formulated for hair removal. Once the wax is applied, gauze is pressed onto it while still warm. When the wax cools and sets, the gauze is ripped away from the skin, taking the hair with it. This is painful, quite painful for some, and the area may stay red and swollen for a day or two. Many women say they get used to it or don't care because they are hair-free for four to six weeks. For some, that is long enough to forget the pain. As for some of us (me included), I'd spend the entire six weeks dreading it.

It is possible to wax at home, but for the full genital area, it makes more sense to use an expert. You can get a bikini line wax where the hair outside the bikini line is waxed, or you can go with a Brazilian wax.

A Brazilian wax is where everything is waxed—anus, outer labia and inner labia. First, you strip down. Once you are in this vulnerable state, the attendant will spread your legs very wide or possibly over your head. From that point, everything is waxed and removed. You will need enough hair to wax off and a final finish with the tweezers. The area will be red, swollen and sore for a few days. The whole process takes about 15 minutes and is only necessary about once a month for a silky smooth area.

Be sure to use a high end salon for the best results. To further enhance the area or for a special occasion, you can have a crystal tattoo, a stenciled design of small clear or colored crystals. The adhesive lasts up to five days or one evening. There are all sorts of patterns including sunbursts, hearts, stars, and butterflies. It might help you forget the ordeal.

Beard Burn

One thing women complain about is men's beards. Men should either grow a full beard or keep it clean shaven. Yes, I know that stubble is trendy and looks sexy, but it is painful. Before you start giving your partner oral sex, take a moment to feel how your facial hair will feel against her sensitive skin. It can hurt! Heavier bearded men may want to shave as soon as fifteen minutes before oral sex. If that's not convenient, you can hold a well positioned towel around the outer lips before you start or drape a towel, one over each leg. If you usually sport a "shadow," you might grow it longer to avoid little stabs to her

Cunnilingus

genital area. If necessary, ask her what she wants.

Setting the Mood

Most women love having oral sex performed on them and many prefer a combination of oral sex and penetration. But some absolutely require oral sex in order to have an orgasm. There is nothing wrong with that. It is perfectly okay to prefer clitoral stimulation to penetration. The point is to let go and have fun, regardless of your personal preferences.

After sharing a bath or shower with your lover so you won't have to worry about unpleasant tastes or odors, start with communication. Men, find out what she likes, and ladies, feel free to tell him. Open up the paths of communication for a great experience.

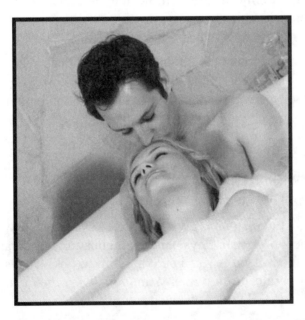

Figure 6: Bathe or Shower Together

Foreplay

Kissing. Kissing is one of the most erotic things you can do to get warmed up. Begin very lightly, then progress to deep French kissing. Deep kissing includes partners rubbing their tongues against each other and over other mouth surfaces. It's teasing, tantalizing and nothing beats it for foreplay. Start slowly, first using just the lips. Don't rush the tongue! Too much tongue too soon can ruin a great kiss.

Women take time to get "in the mood," so, in general, a good sexual encounter should include long and sensual foreplay. Sometimes a quickie can be great, but generally, the more time you spend teasing and not touching, the more fantastic sex will be. Long and sensual foreplay will allow the woman to become engaged in the activity and become properly lubricated.

Communication. There is an axiom that good lovers ask questions, lousy lovers don't. It's difficult to read another's body language even in the best of circumstances, so opening up is the key. Not everything works the same for all women.

For exciting and competent oral sex, feedback is essential. Ask her specific questions and you will get specific answers. Does she want you to go faster, slower, harder or softer? What feels the best: top to bottom or side to side? Should you use circles or long strokes?

As the recipient, give feedback to your lover, which can be physical or verbal. Physical communication might be placing your partner's hand where you want him to lick. It's also fine to ask your partner to stop at any time. In *When the Earth Moves,* author Mikaya Heart poses the question:

> When you ask a friend to come over and take care of your house while you're away, surely you don't expect her automatically to know where everything is? And yet, the first time you go to bed with someone, do you discuss what parts of your body you like to have touched, and how? Do

you even try to explain what turns you on? Do you say what you like and don't like? Well, if not, how can you expect someone to know your preferences, any more than you can expect that person to know where everything is in your house?

As givers and receivers of oral sex, we need to do away with the taboos against talking about what we like and don't like.

Setting the Scene

Gentlemen, for an elaborate lovemaking session of oral sex followed by intercourse, or for oral sex alone, set the scene with candles, flowers and soft music. First, make sure she is comfortable. Spend some time kissing her lips, shoulders, breasts and belly, stroking lightly with your fingertips. Moving down between her legs, gently kiss, blow, stroke and nibble her belly, inner thighs and hips before moving on to the final act.

Erotic massage

Form of Foreplay. Humans need caring physical contact on a daily basis. Before proceeding to oral sex and as an extra added bonus, try erotic massage. The difference between normal massage and erotic massage is that normal massage focuses on the muscles beneath the skin while erotic massage focuses primarily on the skin. With erotic massage, you can calm your lover down from a tough day at work and get her primed for enthusiastic lovemaking. Most likely your erotic massage will arouse her because she will love the intimacy of your actions and because massage releases a great deal of oxytocin, a hormone produced by the posterior lobe of the pituitary gland that stimulates contraction of the smooth muscle of the uterus, into her body. Erotic massage is a great form of foreplay. First she becomes relaxed, and then she will become aroused.

Concentration. Turn off the lights and light scented candles for a relaxing atmosphere. Aromatherapy can be used—

it's lightly scented and neutral, or use traditional scented candles. Put on some sexy, relaxing music and turn off the telephone. You'll want 100% concentration from you and your partner.

Bathe First. Begin with a bath, shower or turn up the juice with a bubble bath. After bathing, she will lie down on the bed or somewhere comfortable. Put a small pillow under her feet, and put another under her legs above the feet. A hand towel under the pillows will protect them from the massage oils. Start at her feet and work up slowly, being careful if she's ticklish. If she is ticklish, use a firmer grip and apply more pressure. The tickling sensation will subside. Moving your thumbs in a circular motion, apply pressure to the balls of her feet. Proceed to the toes and massage each one by lightly squeezing it between your thumb and index finger.

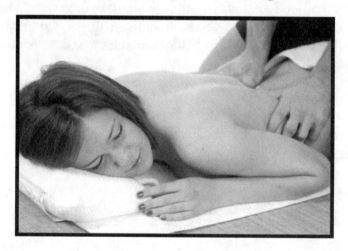

Figure 7: Massage

Neck and Shoulders. The neck and shoulders are common tension spots, so you will want to spend some quality time with these areas. Using a small drop of oil, rub your hands together to make sure they are warm. The hands should be positioned by fanning them out on her upper back. Align your thumbs about an inch away from each other on either side of the spinal cord. Begin the massage using both hands, one on each side of the spine, and rub in a diagonal motion from the spine out. With the tips of your fingers and thumb, gently grip her shoulders and knead the skin. Be careful not to pinch. Go gently, neither hard nor fast. You may also place your hands on either side of her neck and apply a small amount of pressure. Moving your hands in a circular motion—slow and gentle is the rule—work them up behind her ears and back down to her shoulders.

Buttocks. Move down your partner's back and continue circular motions with both hands on either side of her spine. Try light, fluffy touches all over her sides, upper and lower back. Using both hands, one on each side of the spine, repeat rubbing the upper back in a diagonal motion from the spine out. Use quick deep strokes. Move from the upper back to the lower back with the same motion. Then rub her buttocks using the inside of your forearm. Slowly rub each butt cheek in large circular motions. Make a fist and roll your knuckles one by one over the triangular bone at her lower back.

Legs. Moving to her legs, begin at each ankle and knead with your thumbs and fingers all the way up her leg. Don't use a lot of pressure behind the knees. Rub in a circular motion and knead the skin at her thighs.

Head and Face. End the massage at your lover's head and face. Use only the tips of your fingers and gently knead over her temples and head in a circular motion.

Genital Massage

To intensify your massage and your lover's reaction, move to the genital area. She should be on her back for this part of the session, so you can help her roll onto it. You should begin with gentle stimulation of the labia and the whole genital area, *mons veneris* (pubic mound) and vulva. Do not use oils on the vulva; a water based lubricant is recommended. Use light feathery touches and stroke all over her torso and abdomen, the upper thighs and hips. Try cupping your hand over her vulva and hold still for a moment. Press lightly, then begin to move your hand in a modified circular pattern. With light, steady pressure, move the palm of your hand to the outer labia and keep circling.

With the thumb and forefinger of each hand, give a massaging pinch to each outer labia. Stroke the outer lips with both hands, pulling up and down. Using a flat-hand position, press the outer labia in (toward each other) and out. Massage the creases between the inner and outer lips. With a circular motion, massage the thighs working from bottom to top, staying carefully to the sides of the clitoris. It will be too sensitive to touch directly.

Fantasy

Ladies, while your body is being massaged and manipulated by your lover, let your mind wonder freely. Choose a fantasy world all your own. The popular book, *The Secret Garden,* by Nancy Friday, showed that the range of women's fantasies is vast. Don't censor your fantasies. They are a great source for stimulation. Even if you don't find them essential for reaching orgasm, they can still enhance your orgasm. They don't have to be socially acceptable, politically correct, physically feasible, morally admirable, or even legal. Remember, just because you fantasize about something doesn't mean you want to act it out. Fantasies are just that, and nothing more.

4 How to Go Down on a Woman

The Art of Performing Oral Sex

Women love to be teased. When she's breathing heavy, wrap your arms around her hips, cup her buttocks and get to work on her genitals. Don't go after the clitoris like a fireman attacking a fire. Gently spread her legs and kiss her pubic mound. Nuzzle the area for a few minutes, spending time with different parts of her vulva. Begin at the inner part of her thigh, the most tender spot. Lick it, kiss it, and make designs on it with the tip of your tongue. When you are dangerously close to her pussy, glide away. The anticipation will make her tingle.

Lick the crease where her leg joins her vulva. Press your face into her bush and brush your lips over her slit without pressing down on it. Continue licking the area, avoiding a direct hit on the clitoris, until she's very aroused. Open the labia with your fingers. Run your tongue up and down the inside of the slit, between the inner and outer labia. Nibble, with your mouth only, the outer and inner labia. Try kissing the area the way you would her mouth, using your whole mouth, not just the extended tongue. With a soft flat tongue, give her one long 60 second lick. Going slowly is essential. Repeat the process as long as necessary until she begins to melt.

Regularly raise you head and tell her how good she looks, tastes and smells. Be patient; you might be here for a while. If she doesn't respond, try some variations. Let your hands roam. As she becomes more aroused, insert a finger or two in her vagina. Once she is highly aroused, you can stimulate the clitoris more directly.

After she's straining and bucking to get you closer, put your lips right on top of her slit; kiss her gently, then harder. Now use your tongue to separate the lips. When she opens up, run your tongue up and down between the layers of her flesh. Gently spread her legs open with your hands and fuck her with your tongue. Not only does it feel great, but it torments her because she wants the attention directed to her clitoris.

The Clitoris: Step- by- Step

If the clit has hardened enough to peek out of its covering, lick it. If you can't see it, it is still waiting underneath. Move your tongue to the top of her slit and feel her clit. Make it rise by licking the skin that covers it. Lick harder now and press into her skin. Gently pull away the lips and flick your tongue against her clit, whether it is covered by the hood or not.

As she becomes highly aroused, spread her labia and gently kiss and tongue her clitoris. Don't pry back the hood that covers the clitoris unless specifically instructed to or she gives an indication she is ready. Fill your mouth with saliva —never touch or lick the clitoris with a dry finger or tongue. Begin by nipping and biting this tender spot (gently, of course!) and circle it with pursed lips. Sucking like a baby at its mother's breast, use your tongue to gently uncover the clit from its dainty hood. Once you've zeroed in, go around and around with the tip of your tongue, teasing and tickling. Lick and nuzzle the entire area, spending more time on what she likes. Do not spend too

Cunnilingus

long, however, because the area can become desensitized. Bump against the clit, and then change techniques, leaving it alone to throb desperately. Return to kissing her inner thighs, nudging the clit with your face.

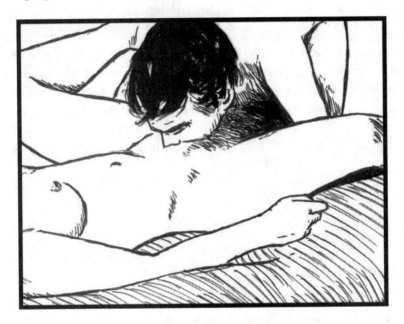

Figure 8: Cunnilingus

Lazily circle the clitoris with your tongue. Lick the shaft from the sides and see if she has a favorite spot. If she rocks her pelvis and moans, you have found the right side. If she jolts or jumps, you have found the right spot, but your technique is too hard.

Quivering is a sign that you should retreat to the sides of the clitoral hood and slow your pace. Lightly flick your tongue over the hood in side-to-side strokes. Not all women enjoy strokes on the clitoral hood because it exposes the sensitive glans. Side-to-side is the best approach, at least in the beginning.

Flatten your tongue and run it over the hood and shaft. Returning to a light flicker, keep going and her response will guide your pressure. Her breathing will change, her skin will flush and her genitals will begin to swell. Her muscles will grow tense. Don't stop because you are getting down to business. If you like, stick a finger in her rear. This should delight her and cause her legs to shudder.

A bucking pelvis indicates orgasm is near; grinding indicates she wants a slow increase in your tongue's tempo. As she approaches orgasm, make your lips into an O and take the clit into your mouth. Suck gently and watch her face for her reaction. If she can handle it, suck harder. If she doesn't like it, return to the tongue flicking. Once you find a pleasing configuration of strokes and the right location, begin to concentrate your efforts there–usually the side of the shaft or even the tip of the clitoris. Proceed by establishing a rhythmic licking that will bring her to the point of orgasm. Develop your rhythm and keep it going. Don't let go! Gradually increase the pressure, but maintain a steady pace. Read her body language. If orgasm is imminent, then don't change anything. Keep doing it–no matter what.

Unlike men, women enjoy strong stimulation while having an orgasm. Keep it going until she tells you to stop. When the tension of rising orgasm lifts her pelvis into the air, move with her and keep your mouth over her clit. Hang on through her orgasm, wrapping your arms around her thighs if necessary. The length of her orgasm can be five seconds to three minutes. It may arrive in groups or waves. Quit when she says so.

Touching Her Emotions

Relax and enjoy. Smile, touch her lightly, hold her if you desire, tell her how beautiful she is and how good she makes you feel, or say nothing and savor the moment. **Your enthusiasm for her goes further than the best of techniques.**

5 Earthquake Status for the Detail Oriented

Mouth, Tongue and Hands

How to Use Your Mouth

Oral fixations are not just for smokers. We are all oral creatures by nature and our mouths are naturally sexual. They talk dirty, look overtly sexual, are strong, wet and warm and trigger mental and physical sexual responses when stimulated. Your mouth is an intimate place on your body right out in the open for all to see.

With your mouth, you can cover the entire vulva area. From this position, nibble the inner and outer lips or the clitoral hood. Suck the clitoris. Don't do it like cock sucking. Try gentle suction with your lips only. Also, you can use suction combined with holding and squeezing the clit for a slow second or two. You can also combine suction with the tongue gently pushing her clit in and out, side to side, or up and down, or circling it. You can gently take her clit in your teeth and hold it, lightly flicking with your tongue.

When your mouth makes full contact with her clitoris, moan appreciatively. It will vibrate her vulva and further excite her. Or try humming "Battle Hymn of the Republic" if you are not shy.

You'll want to keep your mouth nice and clean. When you brush your teeth, brush your tongue as well to keep it smooth and pink. Smile and show off this asset.

How to Use Your Tongue

Getting in Touch with Your Lover. Going down on your lover means getting in touch with your lover—literally. Packages of muscle tissue glands, fatty cells and sensitive nerves, tongues are organs of speech, digestion, and recreation. A mucous membrane covers the tongue while the top surface contains taste buds that are sensitive to touch and food flavors. The surface also houses glands that secrete fluids, including saliva. The brain interprets the flavor of anything we put in our mouths from combinations of the tastes, smells, texture, consistency and temperature. The tongue acts as an erotic messenger to the brain all on its own.

Try this favorite tip: place both hands over the mons creating a diamond shape with the open space between index fingers and thumbs. Rest your nose on your index fingers while you lick the woman's genital area. This position supports your face while you hold open the labia and is easier on the neck.

If you want to know how it feels, wash your hand and lick the palm. This is the most sensitive, ticklish part of your hand, and you can experience how your tongue will feel on your lover's clitoris.

After a few minutes of touching your partner, your mouth will naturally start producing saliva. Keep your tongue moist, without drooling. Your tongue may soon feel dry when you are giving oral sex and this could be irritating to your partner. The tongue should rewet itself or you may try flavored oils if you are still having trouble. Your saliva can flow onto your lover's vulva creating a delightful lubrication. Sometimes,

Cunnilingus

if there is a lot of lubrication coming from her, you can use a towel under her buttocks.

Tongue Strokes and Combinations. Use the tongue strokes that ultimately feel best and get the strongest reaction from your partner. Be sure and keep your upper lip curled protectively over your teeth. Below are listed a few licking techniques to try:

1. Use the tip of your tongue, the blade or underside, the nose, chin, lips and teeth (with caution). Tongue movements can be slow or fast, regular or erratic, firm or soft as the moment requires.

2. If you are having trouble finding your technique, an old standby is to use your tongue as a writing "wand." Start with A and go from there—capitals, lowercase, cursive, secret messages. This method works for those having trouble with technique.

3. Porn star Ron Jeremy has advised in several films that when giving oral sex, a clockwise, counterclockwise, and all-over-the-place approach is more important than focusing solely on the clitoris. Nip with your lips when you change direction.

4. Try swirling your tongue in the space between her hood and mons, and rub the outer labia with flattened fingers. Draw lazy circles around her clit with your tongue.

5. Use a sharp, wide tongue; sharp, round tongue; flat, soft, wide tongue; flat, hard, wide tongue; upside down tongue; or a side curled tongue.

6. Use short, rapid upward strokes, alternated with dipping into her vagina.

7. Lick in circles combined with full open mouthed embraces.

8. Run your tongue back and forth across her inner

lips, then use gentle suction on the lips (labia). Use the same technique on the clitoris.

9. Alternate small, focused circles on either side of the clitoral hood.
10. With your tongue tip, lick in the furrows from top to bottom, pressing in gradually with each stroke.
11. Lick, then plunge your tongue into her vagina; lick and plunge in again.
12. Start with ice cream licks up and down followed with down strokes with your fingertips or flattened thumbs.

How to Use Your Hands

Use your hands to increase her comfort and arousal. You can build her trust by fondling other areas, including breasts, buttocks, thighs and stomach. Insert a finger into her mouth to suck on, run your fingers through or gently pull her pubic hair or lightly tug on the inner or outer labia. Push, pull or rub in circular motion the mons veneris to heighten her intensity. When she is very aroused, squeeze her breasts and nipples.

Ladies, you have the option of showing him where you want him to lick. Make a "V" with your index and middle finger and place it around the designated spot. You may also pull back the skin on your clitoral hood, which will encourage him to lavish attention on your clitoris. Cover it with your finger if it's too sensitive for direct contact.

For the giver, learning to take cues from her body language is imperative. She can move her pelvis closer to you, away from you, either to the right or left, or reposition you completely. There's a risk that she might pull your head down with her hands, grinding upward into your face, or grab your ears or hair. Continue to stimulate and hold her while she climaxes or until she lets you know you can stop. Women's orgasms last much longer than men's, and they can experience waves of pleasure that last several minutes.

Cunnilingus

There is no rhythm that magically makes an orgasm. The best way to help her trigger an orgasm is to pay attention to the location, pressure and timing of your tongue. Communication helps. Let her know beforehand that it's okay to say "harder," "softer," "left" or "right," and "like that," rather than break the mood. Only she can guide you to create her orgasm.

The Etiquette of Receiving Oral Sex

As the woman receiving cunnilingus, it is up to you how much you want to participate. First you give your consent—either out loud or by your body language. You can participate silently or you can be active and give directions on how you want oral sex performed. Some even go so far as to grab their partner's head and direct him to the best spot. Some men find it incredibly arousing when the woman participates in such an active manner. But most women occupy a middle ground. How they react depends upon their degree of arousal and the circumstances.

A soak in a hot tub or a soothing shower before you begin will help to release all your daily tension. At the least, you will want to rinse the area carefully and run your fingers through the pubic hair to pull away any loose stray hairs. Tell or show your partner exactly what you want and have a healthy sense of fun. When you begin receiving oral sex, slow down your internal clock and start savoring each moment.

Breathing

Some women tend to hold their breath during orgasm, so don't forget to breathe. Women who use Tantric practices say that their orgasms are more intense when they use deep breathing techniques. To learn deep breathing, practice when you masturbate. As you touch yourself, inhale deeply into your belly and imagine the breath going all the way down into your pelvis, then back out.

Disappearing Orgasm

Types of orgasm vary. They span from an almost-orgasm, where the woman reaches a peak but never actually releases, to a full blown explosion. Some women occasionally experience a "disappearing orgasm." This is when your energy reaches a peak, but instead of releasing, your orgasm may "implode." A long buildup can slowly fade away to nothing. When this happens, try engaging in oral sex until a peak is reached, then switch to something else. Stop everything for a few moments and take several deep breaths. Relax all your tensed up muscles, breathe from your abdomen, and then let it out. You can return to oral sex or not, but don't try to force orgasm. It usually doesn't work. In fact, stopping and breathing whenever you find yourself getting overly tense can do wonders for your sex life.

Are cleanliness issues holding you back? If you are having trouble getting past a certain point, you and your lover can gradually increase his exposure to your intimate parts until you start to feel more comfortable. Again, a romantic bath or shower can help. You may even begin cunnilingus in the shower.

If you are ashamed of your body, try ambient light or even remain partially clothed. Being partially clothed can add to the forbidden feeling of it all and actually work with your orgasm instead of against it.

The Worst Mistakes

Just as there are a lot of great ways to assist you in oral sex, there are some things you'll want to avoid altogether. *The Master's Guide to Cunnilingus* suggests the following HUGE don'ts for oral sex:

- Don't act like her gynecologist—don't spread her labia so wide she feels like she's getting her annual pap exam; use your fingertips to gently hold back her lips and slip in your tongue.

Cunnilingus

- Don't act like a dog— don't shake your whole head from side to side so that your ears slap against her thighs. Don't lap at her pussy like a puppy lapping up a bowl of water. Keep the tongue loose and relaxed. Don't get sloppy or slobbery and, whatever you do, don't pant!

- Don't act like a leech—don't clamp your mouth around her slit and suck it so hard you give her a welt. Sucking like a vacuum cleaner doesn't feel good, and it might hurt.

- Don't act like an out-of-control Hollywood starlet—drinking and drugs do not mix with cunnilingus. Men need to be able to pay attention and coordinate their tongue action. There is also the additional danger that you might throw up or pass out.

- Don't act like Placido Domingo—don't sing "now I know my ABCs" even if you've opted to trace the ABCs around her clitoris.

- Don't act like Ugly Betty—don't get your braces snagged in her pubic hair. The woman should shave or trim before the session to prevent snaggles, which are painful for her and gross for you.

- Don't act like a preadolescent—don't blow raspberries when going down on her. Some noise is okay, but raspberries, fart sounds or burps don't go over very well.

6 Variations

When it comes to oral sex, there are almost as many variations in sex as there are females that occupy the planet, so there is no "one size fits all." A woman may want clitoral stimulation only while another wants deep vaginal thrusting that pushes against the uterus. Deep thrusting may be too much for another woman who prefers finger penetration to stimulate her prostate. Another woman may prefer a vibrator on her clitoris and penetration at the same time. Some may even prefer breast stimulation, but they are very, very few who can orgasm with breast stimulation alone.

It is possible that, for example, a spinal cord injury can stimulate the development of new triggers for orgasm. Most people, however, will want an orgasm that requires some playing with or manipulation of the sexual organs. Many women desire a combination of oral sex and penetration.

The outer areas of the vulva and opening of the vagina contain more nerve endings than the vaginal canal and respond best to touch and vibration. When performing oral sex, a vibrator can alleviate tongue and jaw cramps, but never put a vibrator directly on the clitoris right away. Because of its extreme sensitivity, always start from the side.

The inner portion of the vagina has fewer nerve endings and responds to feelings of fullness, pressure and rhythm. A vibrator will feel good around the clitoris and the vaginal opening, but only the size, shape and thrusting motion matter once it is inside the vaginal canal.

Women who prefer clitoral stimulation to penetration should not feel ashamed—you share company with a majority of other women. While we are on the subject, let's get rid of some other ideas that are holding us back. It is okay to spurt when the G-spot is stimulated, okay to urinate when you climax, okay to use an electric massager, and it is okay to like anal stimulation. Some women want it all. Let go of old ideas and you will have orgasms in abundance.

Fingering

Men, while you are performing oral sex on your female partner, it is also possible to finger-fuck her. Many women adore the combination.

Use two fingers. One is too skinny and three are too wide so that you can't get deep enough. According to *The Guide for Getting it On,* writer Jay Wiseman noticed that, when lesbian performers in porn movies feel each other up, they almost always use two fingers. When they were asked why, they replied that two fingers simply feel better. Some may enjoy one or three, but most agree that two fingers are best. It also can depend on her state of arousal and sometimes on her menstrual status. Make sure the fingers are wet and slide them slowly inside her. Then start to move a little faster, fucking her rhythmically. Speed up only when her breathing does.

Fisting

Fisting or fist fucking is a sexual activity that involves inserting the hand and forearm into the vagina or anus. Typically, five fingers are kept straight and held as close together as possible, then slowly inserted into a well-lubricated vagina or anus. Vaginal fisting is usually done by women on women because they have smaller fists than men. If you want to try it, please read up before doing so. Anal fisting requires the kind of relaxation beyond the capacity of the average person. Be sure you know what you are doing. Read–*Trust–The Hand Book* by Bert Herrman.

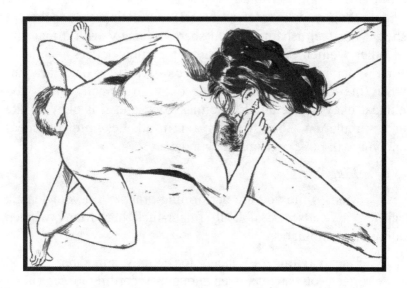

Figure 9: The 69 Position

The 69 Position

The sixty-nine position (69) is when a man gives oral sex to a woman (cunnilingus) at the same time she gives oral sex to him (fellatio). The position can be the female on top on her hands and knees over the man (mouth to genitals), the man on top, or both on their sides. You need to decide which position is the most comfortable position for you. Experiment to see which you like while on the receiving and giving ends. This option overlooks the "kick back and not worry about getting the other person off" attitude that oral sex provides, but sometimes it can be fun. Some couples find it is their favorite way to have oral sex. The simultaneous feelings of sucking and being sucked can be grand.

The 68 Position

The 68 position occurs when the performer lies down, face up, with the receiver on top, also face up, in a head to toe fashion. The position is great for both cunnilingus and anilingus. A pillow should be placed under the giver's head to reduce neck strain. This position allows the performer to use his hands all over his partner's body.

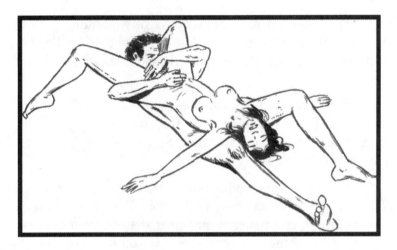

Figure 10: The 68 Position

"Buzzing" or Hummers

Add something extra to a passionate performance. Put your lips around your partner's clitoris or labia and "buzz." A hummer can be performed on both the male and female genitalia. While performing oral sex on your partner, you hum, either a song or just a hum without a rhythm. This, in effect, makes the giver's mouth a vibrator. This vibrator comes with its own built-in lubricant (saliva). The hum effect produces a light, constant vibration that can enhance the oral sex experience. If you tend to the shy side, hum whatever mood music you fancy. The tune isn't important. What is important are the vibrations that will take your partner to new heights of gratification.

You can produce a similar effect by placing a small, powerful vibrator under your jaw. This causes the tongue to vibrate, which can be pleasurable in small amounts. Don't overdo it though. If overused, the process can be numbing for either or both parties.

Afterward

What do you do after you lover reaches her cataclysmic orgasm?

Since her clit will feel very sensitive, holding still for a few moments is a good idea. You may lightly kiss her vulva, but do not begin licking again unless she is multiorgasmic, and she directs you to.

Discover beforehand if she is sensitive about cleanliness. If she is, wipe your face with a damp washcloth before you kiss her on the lips. Some women will like an immediate kiss, but many will not.

Some couples find kissing after sex incredibly erotic; others consider the act somewhat taboo. You may be reluctant because of hygiene issues. Remember that it's your own body, so you have nothing to worry about. If you do have something to worry about, then you should not be allowing someone to go down on you in the first place. If you're concerned about the taste, treat it like an exotic new dish. You won't know if you like it until you've tried it. Try tasting yourself after sex. The bottom line is, it is all personal preference. Do what makes you and your partner feel comfortable. You may decide not to kiss at all or you may decide on a passionate kiss. You'll discover that it intensifies the intimate bond you two already share.

And what about having oral sex after he has already come in your vagina? Some men won't do it; others think there is no problem at all. When a man is heterosexual, he may adhere to an unspoken rule that says a man doesn't perform cunnilingus after he's ejaculated into his partner's vagina. That is ridiculous. It has nothing to do with being homosexual. Whatever you do with your female partner is by definition heterosexual.

Talk to her, stroke her body and caress her breasts. Keep making love quietly until she has come all the way down. A woman requires some sensitivity from her lover in the first few moments after sex.

Clean up afterward. Cunnilingus juices do not age well. Make sure to thoroughly wash all of them off your bodies, brush your teeth and rinse with mouthwash. Don't forget to remove any straggling pubes from your teeth.

7
The Balance of Power: Who Gives and Who Gets (and why not?)!

Reciprocation and Fair Play

As women, it is not uncommon to run into a situation where the man is perfectly happy to receive oral sex from us, but is reluctant to, or flatly refuses, to return the favor. Our response is often intimidation and/or anger. When he won't go down on us, it is easy to feel intimidated. We may feel as if it is our fault or rather, our body's fault, because we are too unattractive, even "dirty."

Sex is all about reciprocation and fair play. Ask your partner why he won't perform oral sex. If he refuses to answer, it may be time to think about changing the relationship. Cowardly behavior is serious, and if your partner is evasive now, chances are you'll never know why. If he is queasy about performing oral sex, then you must know, because your genitals are a very important part of who you are.

Why He Won't Perform Oral Sex

There may be many reasons why he won't perform oral sex.

Unmanly. It is possible that, as the "giver" in a (sometimes considered) taboo act, your lover may be feeling subordinate—not in charge, not "manly." This is the remnant of an old attitude that most of us consciously set aside years ago. In ancient Rome, sexual acts were viewed as acts of submission or control. A man would not perform fellatio or cunnilingus, since that would mean he was penetrated (controlled). It was considered acceptable, however, to receive fellatio from a woman or from a man of lower social status, such as a slave or debtor.

Today there still exists, in some minds, a misconception that labels one partner as passive and the other as active. When a man performs oral sex on his female partner, he could possible interpret it as a sort of power game—one that he is losing. Consciously or subconsciously, he may feel he doesn't deserve respect. In this view, being the "receptive" partner, the receiver, is considered passive, and includes both spreading the legs and opening the mouth. People who eroticize control issues may find that this fuels their arousal, but it can turn others off.

Female Submissive. A woman performing fellatio can be considered responsible for her partner's erection. If she performs oral sex on him to get him hard and remains focused exclusively on his pleasure, then she becomes the submissive one. When he gets on top and begins thrusting—doing what feels good for him—and if she accommodates him regardless of how she feels, she is passive/submissive. Once he comes, she may fake her orgasm. He will doze off and she is once again rendered powerless in the sexual relationship.

In the same way, men are still in charge when they perform cunnilingus—in charge of making the woman have an orgasm. A man may think that since it's "difficult" for a woman to have an orgasm and so easy for him, he will put aside his own pleasure and make sure she has a good time. After all, he doesn't want to feel like a macho jerk.

In fact, a Durex (condom manufacturer) global sex survey reports that 45 percent of American men are more concerned about their partner's enjoyment than their own. Compare that to 32 percent of women.

Individual Interpretation. In actuality, the dynamic of giving and receiving is interpreted entirely by each individual. Neither partner is "in control" of the other. Oral sex, either giving or receiving, is a two-way street where both partners have consented. The man as giver is emotionally exposed because his ability, performance and desire may be judged. The woman as receiver will feel emotionally exposed, but more importantly, she will feel physically exposed as well. She will feel vulnerable with the man's face right up close between her legs.

To establish a comfort level, talk about it beforehand. While some women enjoy the feeling of authority, being in charge and giving directions, others just relax, lie back and let their fantasies go wild. Trust can be cultivated with communication and tenderness.

Sexual Abuse. By removing our feelings of dominance, shame and powerlessness, sexual abuse can become a rare occurrence. Because there are so many taboos that surround open and honest conversation, much less actual intercourse, it makes it easier for people to get away with deviate behaviors. Shielded by a conspiracy of silence, shame forces some to repress any desires that may be considered unacceptable. Repressed desire tends to grow and often becomes dangerous. More openness and honesty could possibly lead to helping disturbed people. Harmless outlets could potentially provide them with more opportunities for help before they harm others.

8 The Tough Part: Understanding Your Female Partner

A Man's Point of View

Different Sexual Experiences

It is commonly known that men and women experience sexuality differently. Can the behavioral differences affected by the production of estrogen and testosterone account for this difference?

Forget penises, vulvas and chromosomes. There is one big difference between the way men and women have experienced sexuality throughout the ages. It is the fact that women get pregnant and men do not. Men do not get knocked up and have to carry a baby inside themselves for nine months, They are not expected to be a child's primary caregiver for the next eighteen years. A lot can be accounted for by this innate knowledge that women have—that with sex comes responsibility, the possibility of another life. We remember this fact in our genes. Couldn't that account for the allegedly less passionate nature of women?

There are many factors that influence how we feel about and act regarding sex. Most factors have to do with cultural roles and expectations, but some actually reflect differences in biology, other than the fact that the woman bears the children. For example, subtle differences in the male and female brain influence different behaviors. If women responded to penises they way they do chocolate, this would be a different world indeed.

So, setting aside for a few pages that women are supposed to be less passionate than men, the feelings men feel are shared by their female partners. You both have feelings that are waiting to be touched, shared and released. From *The Guide to Getting It On:*

> Fortunately, there are a lot of wonderful dimensions to sex besides just huffing and puffing while the bedsprings squeak. Sharing sex with a partner allows you to discover where the different emotions are stored in each of your bodies, where your hopes and dreams are hiding, where the laughter and pain reside, and what it takes to free the fun, passion, and hidden kink. To achieve that level of sharing you have to take the time to know someone, to feel what they are feeling, to see the world through their eyes, and to let a partner discover who you are in ways that might leave you feeling vulnerable. This can be scary.

A Woman's Point of View

Girls may grow up in total ignorance of the existence of their clitoris and vagina. For many girls, it is the use of a tampon that first introduces them to their inner secrets.

There are many factors that influence men's and women's experience of sex. While some have to do with

Cunnilingus

differences in biology, most have to do with cultural roles and expectations. Women are simply brought up differently than men. Requesting oral sex may arouse for her issues of shame about having a man between her legs.

Sexual shame is never too far distant for most women. They feel they should have a perfect body. A woman may also have been taught that sex is dirty, and her genitals are "icky." Influenced by everything from television to parents, women are taught to be ashamed. Many consider oral sex to be more intimate than intercourse. They are self conscious about the way they taste and/or smell, especially when experimenting with a new partner. Most don't like their bodies, even the most beautiful, and they don't want you to get a close look.

Don't underrate the mental aspect of a woman's sexuality. When asking to perform oral sex on your partner or asking her to perform oral sex on you, you have no idea how she will react. If you have a set routine that has not included oral sex to this point, asking for oral sex will take courage, strategy and understanding, especially if your partner is reluctant to perform or receive oral sex. Tell her how much you are looking forward to tasting her, that you love her taste, and that it turns you on. Create space for her to feel comfortable. She might eventually come to love her genitals as much as you do. For a complete sexual experience, you want her to be comfortable sticking her crotch into your mouth.

Combating Sexual Fears

Sexual energy is created on a subconscious level. It is important to go with what our bodies want. Flows of energy may be blocked or allowed to flow, and your partner may have unconscious reasons to block her sexual energy. It may be that women who don't come or don't come easily are not psychologically ready to experience the shocking intensity of what an orgasm can do to them .

Think of how you can ask for oral sex, how you might bring it up. Maybe you can rent a mainstream movie with an oral sex scene in it: *Henry and June*, *Basic Instinct* (the director's cut), *Stiff Upper Lips* (must be British), *Good Will Hunting* and *Kama Sutra*. You might ask (to give or receive) when you are entwined in intimate embrace. Try telling her a story or confessing to a sexual fantasy.

Another way to combat her sexual fears and worries is by masturbation. Masturbation is a natural way of releasing tension and boosting self-esteem. She can masturbate alone or with a partner or have her partner masturbate her for sexual self-reliance. Masturbation is a positive-life-affirming practice that stimulates blood flow to the genitals and keeps them healthy. Masturbation can help a woman learn to orgasm, lose her inhibitions and lose her fear of failing to reach climax.

If oral sex is going nowhere, try switching to other activities such as mutual masturbation or intercourse. Add other stimulation such as masturbating with your fingers, vaginal or anal penetration during oral sex or the sixty-nine position. Getting directly involved may provide the right amount of stimulation or distraction you need. Try sex toys and fantasies and return to her pressure points to increase her arousal. It may take longer than usual when you introduce any new erotic behavior, especially if you are worrying about it.

The Golden Rule of Orgasm for Women is: "The more you do it, the more you'll be able to do it."

9 More Fun: Varying Your Positions

There are many excellent positions for oral sex. Oral sex can be performed from virtually any and every angle, but some are more comfortable than others for her and easier on the man's neck. The main question to ask is, is it comfortable after 5, 10 or 15 minutes? You just have to find the one that suits you and your partner the best.

Cunnilingus Positions

Classic

The classic position is the female on her back with her legs spread, and the man lying on his stomach. This provides the best access to the entire genital area and allows the woman to lie back and relax. It also allows the most options: for penetration, anilingus, making use of pressure points and other tricks. If it becomes tiresome for the man, she can change positions easily. She can adopt variations or place a pillow under her buttocks and allow the man to prop himself up on a pillow as well.

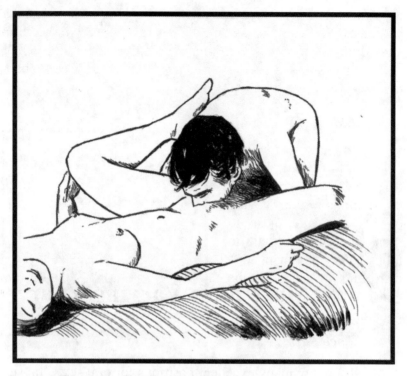

Figure 11: Classic Cunnilingus Position

Doggie style

As in intercourse, doggie style is the woman kneeling on all fours with the man behind her. In oral sex, the female's genitals are licked from behind. This gives good access and feels good. Because she has to maintain this posture, however, the relaxation factor (for the woman) is not as good as the classic position.

Kneeling

The man kneels in front of the female while she stands. This is a great way to begin, but it is tough on his knees, and she can't relax. You can move from this position to the classic.

Seated

It is possible for the female receiver to sit on the edge of

Cunnilingus

the bed while her partner kneels on the floor with pillows under his knees. She can also sit in a chair and scoot to the edge to allow him easier access. Her arms can go over the armrests. For that matter, she can sit on the edge of anything: a bed, chair, table or even the swimming pool.

Sideways

In the sideways position, the female lies on her side. The man can use her thigh as a pillow, lying on his left side, nose to mons or right side, chin to mons. Very pregnant women find this one of the most comfortable of all positions.

Face Sitting

The female doesn't actually sit on the man's face, but kneels on either side of his head and squats with her genitals over his mouth. This is a good position for her to control the action. She can also

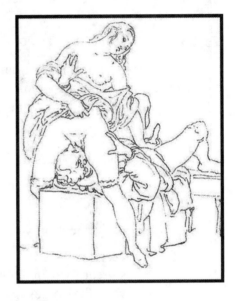

Figure 12: Face Sitting

Drawing by Francisco Hayez (1791-1882) Italy

face either direction, with her buttocks on the man's chest or reverse her position and have access to his genitals. Also called "sitting on his face," the receiver sits on the giver's face and pushes into it with her genitals.

Hummer

A "hummer" is where the giver hums or sings at the same time as he is performing oral sex. In effect, this turns his mouth into a vibrator. It is better than a mechanical vibrator because he has a built in lubricant (saliva).

Autocunnilingus

The kicker of all variations on position may be the autocunnilingus position–or performing oral sex on yourself. This may be possible for extremely flexible women, like contortionists or dancers, but most of us aren't going to want it anyway. If you want to learn, there is information in books and on the internet.

Variations

Here are some more variations a person can try while performing oral sex on a woman:

1. Raise one of her legs and bend it over your shoulder or to her chest.
2. Place both legs over your shoulders.
3. Have her lie on her back with her knees pressed to her chest.
4. Put her feet ON your shoulders.
5. Keep her legs flat (in the classic position). This is great for women who like to flex their thighs when they orgasm.
6. Place pillows under her buttocks to raise her legs or place a pillow behind her back. You can put a pillow under your chest for added comfort.
7. Try licking from a right angle when she is on her back.
8. Wrap your arms under her thighs and toward you over her hips. From this position, you can open or massage her labia.
9. Grasp and lift her buttocks, supporting her hips with your hands.

Remember, all these positions are good ones. You just need to find (with your partner) what works best for the two of you.

Positions for the Disabled or Injured

The disabled and injured do not have to be denied the joys of oral sex. Never consider a disabled person asexual.

There are different kinds of disability. A third of women with diabetes can't achieve orgasm. Paraplegic and quadriplegic women's sexual function may be impaired. It is possible, however, to gain sensitivity in other areas to make up for what has been lost. A great scene in the movie, *Coming Home*, with Jon Voight and Jane Fonda, showed just how hot oral sex can be for a paralyzed man.

Here are some positions that can help:

1. If she can't walk, loop her legs over your biceps.
2. Use props and bolster pillows to attain the right position.
3. Cunnilingus strains the neck muscles, so beware of injuries to this area. If the man has a neck injury, choose positions that support the head. For example, a sideways 69 or woman on top using her thigh as a pillow can work. He can also sit backward in a high-backed chair while she's on the kitchen counter, for example.
4. For back injuries, use pillows under the knees, between the knees or to cushion whoever is feeling awkward or hurting.

10 Don't Stop There: Taking It to the Next Level

Oral sex, in and of itself, can be fantastic, but you also have the option of taking it a step or two further. If you want to intensify a woman's pleasure, there are other ways to manipulate her.

G-Spot Stimulation

One way to increase your partner's enjoyment is to finger fuck her at the same time you perform oral sex. By inserting one or more fingers, you can add a special touch by stroking her G-spot.

Both women and men have a ring of spongy erectile tissue surrounding the urethra (where urine leaves the body). The spongy erectile tissue is actually the periurethral sponge (or urethral sponge), or commonly in women, the G-spot or G-spot prostate. In the female, the urethra is a tube about two inches long located inside the vagina, running from the bladder to the

Cunnilingus

urethral opening. The urinary canal, prostate, vagina and clitoral body are all close together. Located on the front wall of the vagina, toward the belly button, roughly two inches inside the vagina, the G-Spot is an integral part of the clitoral system. It can be felt through the walls of the vagina. When not aroused, the sponge is relaxed and difficult to feel. Once aroused, the sponge swells and hardens.

To stimulate the G-Spot, insert one or two fingers about one to two inches inside the vagina and press up, toward her belly button. Curve your fingers and stroke in a stiff "come hither" motion. Combine a good session of cunnilingus with your finger stimulating her G-spot, and you will create a masterful oral sex scenario. Her response will often be an unbelievable orgasm, one more intense and fulfilling than one with clitoral stimulation alone.

This area also responds pleasurably to rhythmic massage. Oral sex and vibrators can be used together for excellent G-spot stimulation. Dildos and vibrators that are firm plastic with a curve at the tip are excellent for this purpose. A heavy duty vibrator should be pressed against the vulva and angled slightly upwards.

With your head "down there," it is convenient to stimulate the G-spot with fingering while performing oral sex. And while all this is going on, don't forget to keep licking.

Squirting

The intense sexual arousal from the combination of oral sex, deep penetration and direct G-Spot stimulation may cause the female partner to ejaculate. Female ejaculation is a gush of clear fluid from the urethral sponge. Produced by the 30 or more tiny prostrate-like glands surrounding the G-Spot (called periurethral glands), female ejaculate is an alkaline fluid similar to male prostatic fluid, without the semen. This makes sense: homologous to the male prostate gland, the G-Spot is usually highly sensitive. When viewed as a single sex organ, the ceiling of the vagina is the floor of the urinary canal. Pressing up into the roof of the vagina to stimulate the female prostate is similar to stimulating the male prostate from inside the anus, which can trigger male ejaculation. Female ejaculation may borrow urine from the bladder but it is not urinating. Stroking the G-Spot gets these glands engorged and primed. The longer you stroke, the juicier they get. The contractions of orgasm can force out the fluids in a gush of liquid called ejaculation, called "squirting" and "spurting."

Ejaculating

Most women in our world don't know how to ejaculate. Female ejaculation is barely acknowledged and reluctantly accepted by many people even today, including physicians.

Western society has ignored female sexuality for centuries. Ejaculation was known in ancient times, and was even mentioned by Aristotle. It is commonly acknowledged in some present day cultures. The South Pacific Trobriand Islanders described female ejaculation to Western anthropologists who, because of their ignorance, assumed they were speaking of urination. The Batoro people of Uganda don't consider a woman eligible for marriage until she can spray the wall from her G-Spot. The older women of the tribe teach her how to do so.

Today, in our culture, G-Spot stimulation and squirting has taken hold, to some extent. Numerous women and their partners find it exciting, while others find it disconcerting. While some squirt a few teaspoons, others may squirt a lot—one cup or more. If you object to getting a squirt of liquid in the face, let your partner know that you prefer she abstain from spraying you in the face.

If, as the female, you want to learn (or at least try) squirting, you can learn how by bearing down at the moment of orgasm. Some female ejaculators who do sexual performances admit to drinking a giant bottle of water before going onstage or in front of a camera.

Nonetheless, many women apparently have never

Cunnilingus

ejaculated and some have ejaculated from the beginning of their sexual activity. While some women can teach themselves how to do it, there are others who try to learn without success. And some women could care less. The amount varies as well. While some squirt teaspoons others just flood.

Often, women in their 40s begin ejaculating when they never had before. In her 40s, a woman may simply be at an age where she is more open and relaxed, mentally and physically, and more receptive to "letting go." She may be more incontinent, and squirting is therefore easier.

Squirting is also associated with the practice of fisting (see *Glossary*).

Most women find that once the G-Spot is firm with arousal, touch and vibration are delightful. But others dislike the sensation, often because it is accompanied by an urgent feeling of having to pee. This can be too intense for many women. A woman may feel she is actually urinating when she is ejaculating, and ejaculation is often misdiagnosed as urinary stress incontinence.

Although the ducts of the periurethral glands empty into the urethral canal, ejaculation is not urinating. The chemical composition of fluid is different from urine, although it contains a small amount of the same substances. Researchers who have analyzed ejaculatory fluid say it is different than urine, although it may include a small portion of urine if a residual amount was retained in the urethra.

Female ejaculation is perfectly fine and not an aberration. To fear it is a relic of our religious disgust with bodily fluids.

If you are afraid of making a mess, give yourself permission to experiment. Try stimulating yourself immediately after you have peed, while still sitting on the toilet, or use a plastic sheet on the bed. You have the right to determine for yourself what feels good and to do it, and most of your fears are unfounded.

Call it spunk, ejaculate, spurt, drool, or pee. If it feels good, go for it. A towel or rubber sheet on the bed will help when you let go.

Anilingus

What is it?

What is the last part of your body to get any attention? Many people end up going through life without discovering the anus as an important erogenous zone. Anilingus and cunnilingus go together like sado and masochism.

Rimming or anilingus is kissing, caressing or penetrating your lover's anal opening with your tongue. Oral sex provides a perfect way to introduce anal play. It can add a whole new dimension to oral sex. Some say that there is nothing as arousing as anal sex to give, and many love to receive it. The fact that anal sex is considered dirty and usually taboo probably enhances the feeling of excitement.

Anilingus is a sensitive subject with most women. Go slowly and pay careful attention to the person you are penetrating. It is probably not a good idea to introduce it until your partner is highly aroused.

Even a little anilingus can be highly erotic. The area is packed with sensitive nerve endings, which makes it highly sensitive to a gentle, playful loving touch by the fingers, lips and tongue. The pelvic floor muscles lie beneath the surface of the anal area. They play an important role in sex and contract during orgasm. Using a sex toy, finger or tongue to massage or insert into the anus stimulates the pelvic floor muscles and heightens overall erotic sensations.

Technique

To stimulate a woman's butt when you are performing oral sex, insert one finger just past the sphincter muscle. Do not slide it all the way in and out. It is preferable if there is a slight tugging movement. Begin with a flat finger or fingers and press lightly on the opening. Hold your finger there as you increase

Cunnilingus

the pressure a little. Then move your flattened fingers in a circular motion, massaging and caressing the opening's base. If she wants you to go further, slowly slide your finger in to the first joint (about one inch) and wait for the contracted muscles to relax. Once relaxed, if she wants more, slide the finger in further and then pull out. Go in and out very slowly. You may also add more fingers. Take your time and listen for cues and instructions. Read her body language. This may be all it takes for her to reach orgasm.

If you (and she) want to go even further, with her anus in full view, kiss and lick her butt checks toward the inside, working closer into the furrow. Make first contact with her anus by licking the entire furrow from top to bottom with a flattened tongue. With soft lips, kiss the anus over and over. Press a flattened tongue against the opening and hold it at first, then slowly start to move up and down. With the tip of your tongue, lightly lick in a ring around the rim of the opening (thus, "rimming").

The anal area does not have the natural lubrication of the vagina, so do not rely on your saliva alone. Use a thick water-based lubricant. Anal penetration can hurt, so be sure and use enough lubricant, and go very slowly. Make sure she is relaxed at every turn. Flavored lubricants are an option, but they taste awful and are packed with sugar. They are not an option for diabetics or people who don't tolerate the effects of sugar. If they get inside the vagina, they will most likely cause a yeast infection. Also, beware of lubricants that advertise "anal ease" because they can numb the tongue and anus.

You can further spice things up during cunnilingus by inserting an index finger in her butt and your thumb in her vagina.

For an added dash, you can add anal sex toys. The best have a flared base so they cannot be drawn into the anal opening, a real danger since the anal muscles contract and squeeze on their own. It may be hard to control them. A lost toy might not come out without a trip to the hospital, so buy safe toys and don't experiment with vegetables. You can also use vibrators, dildos and butt plugs.

Not everybody feels comfortable with the thought of kissing or licking their lover's anus, or with having it done to them. The man may be accidentally introduced to anilingus during cunnilingus, since the bottom of the vaginal entrance is close to the anus. Sometimes, a lick meant for the lower vagina slips further down than intended. The recipient may experience an unexpected thrill and perhaps decide to explore anilingus further.

Anilingus is not wrong or abnormal. Not too long ago, oral sex was considered a disgusting perversion and was outlawed in many states. These days, three quarters of Americans say they had performed it on a lover and had it performed on them. Some day the same might be said for anal sex.

Fun Without Fear

Although anilingus is incredibly pleasurable to some people, it provides its own special concerns. It is not a totally safe practice without some protection. Possible infections include hepatitis A, anal herpes, anal warts, and possibly viruses such as HIV. If you enjoy unprotected sex, oral or otherwise, on a first date, then any partner is high risk. The only sure prevention is a truly monogamous couple where each is confident that neither has hepatitis, HIV nor intestinal parasites, or abstinence.

The digestive tract is home to millions of bacteria that assist in digestion and contact may expose the giver of anilingus to these bacteria. The micro-organisms get incorporated into the stool and can be found in and around the anus. Although they help with digestion, they might also cause infection. E. coli is the most notable of these micro-organisms. If E. coli comes into contact with the vagina or urethra, the woman may develop a vaginal infection or a urinary tract infection (cystitis or bladder infection).

Other micro-organisms (other than E. coli) that can spread during oral-anal contact are:

Shigella and Salmonella, which cause food poisoning. These micro-organisms cause acute and vicious diarrhea. Someone with mild symptoms may transmit the infection to someone else who develops severe symptoms.

Intestinal parasites, notably Giardia lamblia and amoebas, both which cause diarrhea.

Viruses, notably HIV and the one that causes Hepatitis A. HIV typically spreads through blood-to-blood contact. Anal tissue bleeds easily, particularly in the estimated 1/3 of American adults who have hemorrhoids. (Varicose veins of the anal canal sometimes cause pain, but frequently do not. Affected individuals may not know they have them.) If HIV contaminated blood enters the mouth of someone who has a minor injury—bleeding gums, for example—the infection might be transmitted.

Enemas and careful washing eliminate most of the risk. Monogamous couples who practice careful anal hygiene are at extremely low risk of causing infection or illness.

Fecal Contact. Because the anus is intimately involved in defecation, may people assume that oral anal contact must involve contact with feces. This is a distinct possibility, even with careful wiping. Traces of fecal material may cling to the anus and the skin around it. By practicing careful personal hygiene, you can minimize this exposure. Jack Morin, Ph.D., author of *Anal Pleasure and Health*, states that the anus, anal canal and rectum usually contain little stool. Most fecal material is stored above the rectum in the descending colon. When the stool moves into the rectum, you feel the urge. It then passes out of the body fairly quickly. When you feel no urge to defecate, there are only trace amounts of stool in the rectum, anal canal and anus. These traces can easily be washed out.

If you take prudent precautions, anilingus can be a safe practice. Be careful to avoid getting bacteria from the anus into her vulva or vagina by going back and forth from her clit to her butt. This can result in a nasty infection. If you have been performing anilingus, be sure to wash and rinse your face and mouth before going back to cunnilingus. The standard recommendation is that anything that comes into contact with the anus should not touch the vulva or vagina afterward.

Cleanliness. Cleanliness is the number one concern. Thoroughly wash the area in and around the anus with soap and water before any sexual encounter involving the area. Taking a long shower or bath before is recommended and has the added benefit of relaxing the participants. You also can begin anilingus or oral sex combined with anilingus in the shower where both of you are squeaky clean. Showering together is great sensual foreplay.

If your female partner is comfortable with enemas, you can do that before showering. An enema, though not necessary, is an extra margin of hygiene safety. Enemas rinse the rectum and anal canal, removing most traces of fecal material. Today, they are easy to use, especially the disposable enemas available over the counter from pharmacies.

For high-risk anal sex, i.e. first time partners, non-monogamous relationships, etc., use dental dams, plastic wrap, or cut open condoms to use over the anal area prior to licking or tonguing.

Dental Dams. A dental dam is a thick sheet of latex rubber that works like a condom, acting as a physical barrier between the anus and the mouth. For penetration, you can use gloves and finger cots. Using these barriers may feel awkward at first, but like condoms, they can be used during anilingus easily with a little practice and a sense of humor. They are readily available at most pharmacies. You may also buy unlubricated condoms or latex gloves and cut them into flat sheets. In a pinch, you can use plastic food wrap. To heighten pleasure, massage a little sexual lubricant into your lover's anus before applying the dam.

Cunnilingus

After anilingus without a dam, be sure to rinse your mouth with an antiseptic mouthwash, or at the very least, water.

Anilingus Positions

What are the best positions for anilingus? If it is a part of cunnilingus, you will want to get into the best position for both. There are plenty of options.

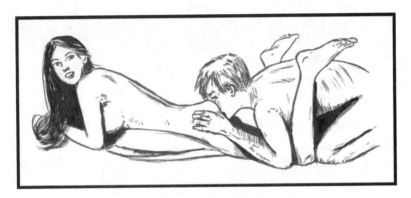

Figure 13: Anilingus

Knees and Elbows. The receiver assumes the rear entry position (doggie style) while her lover kneels or squats behind her, gently spreading the cheeks to expose the vulva and the anus. This is one of the easiest positions because you can see everything clearly as you lick and stroke. You can part the hair to make everything more accessible.

Standing, Bent Over. The receiver stands and bends at the waist while the giver kneels, sits or squats behind.

Lying Supine. The receiver lies on her back, legs bent, and knees drawn up to the chest or apart. The giver squats or lies on his stomach. Place a pillow under the recipient's hips, raising the anus and allowing for easier access to the vulva and the anus.

It's possible for the receiver to lie on her stomach with pillows under her hips. The anus is accessible, but the clitoris is harder to reach.

The sixty-nine position is also possible, but it requires some physical flexibility. Nonetheless, many people enjoy this position for cunnilingus and anilingus.

Some Final Tips

TAKE IT SLOWLY! Unless your partner specifically requests that you go faster, approach with care and go slowly. Work your way toward the anus by massaging, kissing and licking her lower back, thighs, hips and buttocks. A slow approach builds her anticipation and heightens the eroticism of anilingus. It is better to spend time massaging and caressing the external butt and anal parts if you want to increase your partner's enjoyment.

Vary Your Technique. Discover what your partner likes. You can make your tongue thin like a finger or wider like a penis or dildo. Use the flat of your tongue and press it against the anus. Use the tip of your tongue and wiggle it around the anus, slip it inside and move it in and out. Or wiggle it around in circles. When she groans and moans and pushes her butt in your face, stay with it for a while. Then you can start tongue-fucking. Moan and if she moans in return, it will vibrate the tongue.

If you use sex toys, in and out movements are best served by a dildo, while staying stationery works best with something like a butt plug.

Intense power is drawn when lovers wholeheartedly accept each other. Anilingus involves acceptance of an area that is not normally acceptable. Performing anilingus on your lover says "I love all of you – every part." The receiver says: "I'm totally yours. No part of me is off limits to you." This level of mutual acceptance is a powerful turn on.

11

Double Dare: Fantasies and Bondage

Fantasizing

Brain Largest Sex Organ

What is the largest sex organ in our bodies? Many suggest that the brain occupies that position. The brain plays an integral part in orgasm. Without being "in the mood," there is no way to achieve orgasm without it. The brain can also manufacture fantasies that can enhance and bring on your orgasm.

Fantasizing freely is truly one of the joys of oral sex. As the receiver, you can choose to lie back, be lazy, let your partner do all the hard work, and let your fantasies run wild.

Fantasy, or at least the dirty kind, the kind that gets you off, is often not a big part of many women's lives. Most of us grew up reading romantic love stories that were based on being pretty and sweet enough to catch the handsome prince. An entire fantasy might consist of imagining a future together, including the silverware pattern. Romance, not sex, was the stuff dreams were made of.

Some romance is great—especially when sex is involved—but those kind of fantasies are not very conducive to the down-and-dirty thoughts that help most women achieve orgasm.

The sexual revolution moved things along quite a bit. With more freedom to experiment and become sexually fulfilled came reality. Fantasies devoted to visions of romantic love and fairy tale obsessions based on how beautiful we can look in order to capture the mythical prince were abandoned. They are a hindrance to sexuality and orgasm. That's why too many women spend their lovemaking concerned about how they look or trying to hold their stomachs in instead of enjoying the act. These days, happily, more and more women are learning to enjoy the hot sexual fantasies more typical of men.

Are Fantasies Sick?

You may secretly believe your fantasies are too sick or kinky to use without guilt, but there is a long list of sexual scenarios that are quite popular and harmless. Some of the fantasies that people enjoy are: playing doctor, being made to perform sexually against your will, rape scenes, being punished or humiliated, getting strip searched; having sex with a baseball or soccer team or other gang bang scenes, sex with relatives, and sex with angels, to name a few. The endless list reflects our individual needs and experiences. There is no need to pass judgment on the morality of fantasies. Many times, probably most of the time, fantasies contain scenes we would never perform in real life and probably wouldn't enjoy if we did. A creative mind demands a limitless field of possibilities.

Your fantasies may be full of paradoxes. A dominant person may become submissive; a submissive person can become dominant in her fantasies. A gay person may be straight, and a straight person may experience homosexual or bisexuality. A feminist may fantasize rape. Control freaks build

Cunnilingus

scenes of bondage. For some women, the image of being totally helpless is a psychic vacation—a rest from always running the show. In fact, the best clients of S&M parlors are the big power brokers in business and government.

In our fantasies, we can imagine things that we never intend to experience in real life. We play roles in fantasies—all of the roles: rapist and rapee, the woman and the man, master and slave. We can explore the dark corners of our minds or have sweet and light romantic fantasies as long as we thoroughly enjoy the orgasm that comes with it.

We can use sexual fantasies to our advantage in other ways. If a new sexual experience is potentially scary, turn it into pleasure by fantasizing. Use your imagination, read erotica, listen to hot audiotapes and watch erotic movies to enhance your imagination.

In your fantasy, you don't have to be politically correct, faithful to your partner or even have safe sex. Fantasies aren't real and using them to get off doesn't mean you want them to necessarily come true. Your head is an erotic safe place. Don't feel guilty if you want to have sex with strangers in your head—any number of them.

How to Fantasize

Most X-rated pornography is geared toward the male market. Very often women miss out having visual references for sex that can fuel fantasies. Women seldom have detailed sexual conversations with friends and lovers or share hot talk about sex. Nude photos of men, women or couples making love might be interesting or even pleasing, but it is not necessarily what a woman fantasizes about. Nonetheless, women can become turned on by porn just like men.

Any woman can learn to explore her own mind for sexual ideas and weave them into erotic stories that will intensify her orgasm.

Dare to develop and expand your fantasy world. Replay

a hot sexual experience in your mind; combine different sexy moments from different sexual encounters and read books and magazines. Watch movies and porn on TV. If the plots bore you, fast forward to the good parts. Look for specific images and ignore the plotting and characterization, which will be pretty poor. The sight of couples endlessly thrusting and pounding in every position can become repetitious and boring. Even the worst porn, however, can contain something that triggers your imagination.

You can also learn to enjoy phone sex. Speaking of intimate matters may be difficult at first, but practice can lead to some spicy conversations. Try to keep reality from ruining the experience for you—the reality that it is probably some bedraggled, not-very-attractive person on the other end of the line.

Some couples enjoy talking dirty while having sex, which is fine if both partners enjoy it. However, if a partner can't perform without hearing dirty words, it could strike his or her partner as almost fetish-like and perhaps degrading.

Although it's not a requirement and doesn't always have to occur, fantasies can lead lovers to explore whimsical sex roles. If you decide to participate in role-playing, there are some basic rules you will want to follow.

Establish a red light and green light, *i.e.*, where to touch and where to not touch. As you touch various parts of the body, you can give verbal cues of one to ten. One means softly; increasing the number means to turn up the volume.

There are some fairly simple soft-porn fantasies you can act out, if you wish. For one, there is dressing up for sex—the traditional garter belt, bra and high heels—but there are literally thousands of other outfits to wear and fun games to play.

What Men Can Do

Men, you can try putting a sliver of ice in your mouth and let it melt while licking your partner on her neck, nipples,

Cunnilingus

vulva and clitoris. Or you can let small drops of water fall on these erogenous zones. You can use the physical sensations caused by silk, velvet, fake fur, rubber, leather, ice, a hot cup of tea, a feather or a vibrator. Try a blindfold to increase the sensations of touch. If you've never seen the movie *Nine-and-a Half Weeks*, then rent it for some great fantasy ideas.

You can alternate kisses with licks and have her describe the sensations. Use ice and hot tea to warm and cool your mouth alternately; then use your mouth on your partner.

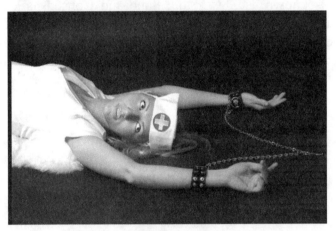

Figure 14: Light Bondage and Role Playing

Bondage, Sadism and Masochism
BDSM

BDSM (Bondage/Sadism/Masochism) describes a number of related patterns of human sexual behavior. The practice of bondage and its cousins can be used during oral sex.

The simplest form of BDSM—gently restraining the wrists and ankles—is possible as are many variations on this theme. The major subgroupings of BDSM are:

Bondage and Discipline (B&D);

Domination and Submission (D&S); and

Sadism and Masochism (S&M).

If these practices were performed in a neutral atmosphere of nonsexual content, they would likely be considered unpleasant and undesirable and probably even abusive. Pain, physical restraint and servitude are traditionally inflicted on persons against their will and to their detriment. In BDSM, however, these activities are engaged in with the mutual consent of the participants, and typically for mutual enjoyment. The emphasis is on *informed* consent and safety is important. Safety is known as SSC (Safe, Sane and Consensual). Some prefer the term RACK (Risk Aware Consensual Kink), placing more emphasis on acknowledging the fact that activities are potentially risky. Both terms refer to the fact that all participants acknowledge and accept some level of risk.

Safety Tips

Role Playing

Rules. If you and your partner decide to participate in role-playing or engage in light bondage, be sure to follow these basic rules for safety:

1. If a body part feels numb or goes to sleep, untie it immediately.
2. Never tie anything around your partner's neck.
3. Anticipating fires, earthquakes or visits from mom and dad, keep a flashlight and a pair of scissors and/or handcuff key ready.
4. Never leave a person for long and check back often. You are legally responsible for injuries.
5. Establish a safe word or gesture which means to stop and honor it without question.
6. Don't confuse for a second real abuse (someone who enjoys beating the crap out of people) with bondage. In heavy bondage, there are established rules and etiquette that keep participants from getting seriously hurt.

Cunnilingus

In spite of the ongoing bad rap pornography receives, there are large numbers of people who enjoy sharing sex related entertainment, including porn movies, x-rated videos, sex books, calling party lines, exploring fetish wear and buying adult toys. Governments and religions may try to repress the primal urge for sex, but no matter how much they try, they will never succeed. If you want to explore these alternatives to plain vanilla sex, then by all means do so.

Sex Toys

Certain women enjoy some form of penetration during oral sex. It is possible to penetrate your partner using sex toys while also performing oral sex. Your head must be at the right angle, and you must have ample room. Use your fingers, a dildo or a vibrator.

Dildos and Vibrators

A vibrator or dildo can be held in a stationery position while you lick. They come in all shapes and sizes- firm (plastic or silicone) or softer (jelly rubber and Cyberskin). Does she prefer long, medium or short? Bumpy or smooth? Curved or straight? There are as many personal preferences as there are shapes, sizes and colors.

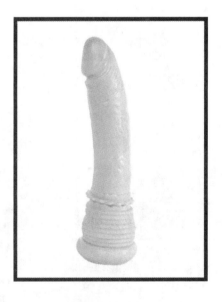

Figure 15: Dildo

Dildos. A dildo is anything used for penetration that doesn't vibrate. They come in penis shapes, partial or whole shapes with smooth curves or bumpy ribs. There is even a blow-up dildo attached to a hand held bulb to enlarge them once they are in place. A dildo performs like your husband's penis, with the exception that it is always available and always hard. It never grows tired and cranky, never becomes soft, never gets diseased (wash thoroughly or use condoms or both) and never gets in the way. Buy several in different shapes and sizes for an exciting variety.

Vibrators. Vibrators provide strong, steady stimulation. They come in many shapes and sizes with variations of speed and motion. They can be used to penetrate the vagina or not. Do not use porous models, as they can retain bacteria. Use them with condoms.

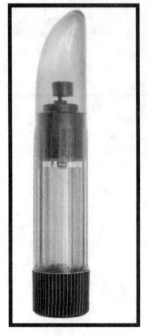

Figure 16: Simple Plastic Vibrator

Some vibrators with a shaft can be inserted into the vagina. Some vibrate, some pulse, some come with multiple speeds and dials. With a vibrator, a woman can make up for years of sensory deprivation and many women swear by them (and get off with them).

To use a vibrator during oral sex, have your partner lie down on a pillow with a slimline vibrator placed on top of it. It should settle between the butt cheeks so it rests against the body. Once she is comfortable, turn on the vibrator and begin oral sex. The combination of these amazing sensations will send your lover through the roof!

Fingers

If you use your fingers instead of a sex toy, make sure your hands are clean, fingernails trimmed and smooth, no tiny cuts or hangnails. Latex gloves give a firm, slippery sensation.

Cunnilingus

You can start with one finger and add more. Move in and out with a thrusting rhythm following the natural curve of her body. Try beginning with just a little and ask her what she wants you to do next. Some like the thrusting action. You can lick and pump simultaneously.

Sex Toys and Safety

Use common sense when playing with sex toys. Using vegetables (carrots, cucumbers, etc.) is popular, and some vegetables work, but be careful. Do not use a plastic bottle without a lid as a penetration device. It may create suction, and you will be unable to get the bottle out. Do not use anything with sharp edges or anything made of glass which might break. Do not use anything round, like a ball, which could be difficult to remove later.

Tongue Piercing

A simple metal ball placed in the center of the tip of the tongue by piercing can add a new dimension to any oral sex. The ball can give extra firm stimulation right when and where it is needed. Practice using it on your hand so you can learn to control the type of sensation and pressure it delivers.

Curious Facts about Oral Sex

Oral sex has a rich and varied history. Some interesting facts are:

1. Oral sex was illegal in Georgia until 1998

2. There is an alcoholic cocktail named the "Cunnilingus."

3. The Chinese Empress Wu Hu demanded visiting dignitaries lick her clit before any discussion took place. That's how she got her name—Wooo Hooo!

4. The Jehovah's Witnesses say any form of oral sex is "against nature" and therefore sinful.

12 Advanced Intimacy: Some Things You Might Not Want to Think About

Is your goal in having oral sex orgasm or simple pleasure? Is it the main course or just the warm up for penetration?

Some men think they have not pleased a woman unless she has an orgasm, but oral sex doesn't always have to lead to orgasm. Oral sex can be about simply delighting your lover in a new and exciting way. As women, we can demand orgasm, but as a rule, it is better to be more flexible. Using oral sex as a teaser to the main event is also a fun way to go. The **very best** thing you can do is to let yourself go, have fun, and men—you should want her dearly.

Menstruation

Oral Sex and a Woman's Period

About once a month, women bleed around three teaspoons of liquid. Some lovers don't mind mixing oral sex and menstrual blood. Others do. The decision is up to you, but you should be aware that you are exchanging bodily fluids that could turn out to be lethal. You both should be in full agreement about oral sex during this time and should both be comfortable with the decision. Others, both men and women, find it just outright unappealing.

In Islamic literature, there are only two forms of sex that are explicitly prohibited between married couples. Anal sex is one. The other is sex during the menstrual cycle. Although it is not specifically mentioned, some Islamic authorities consider it unclean because of "objectionable" fluids emitted during intercourse that come in contact with the mouth. Other authorities say there is no evidence to forbid it in Islamic literature. Once again, follow your conscience and follow your own desires. If you want to do it, then there is no scientific reason not to.

Talk about it with each other. Women who have grown up in households that weren't supportive of biological processes may feel unlovable or unattractive during this time. Do you want to perform oral sex during her period and does she want you to? Those are the only questions that need to be answered.

Early Onset Menstruation

The onset of menstruation in young women is occurring at steadily earlier ages in the Western world. This is usually attributed to better nutrition, but it may actually be caused by poorer nutrition. There is strong evidence that early onset may be related to body fat. As you can't help hearing on today's news, the people in Western societies are getting fatter, particularly in the United States. In order to have a menstrual cycle, a girl needs 17% body fat and 26% body fat in order to ovulate. Our penchant for junk food and a sedentary lifestyle is lowering the age where we reach those percentages. It is also likely that the artificial hormones in meat and dairy products contribute to younger onset of menses.

Pregnancy

Can you perform or receive oral sex during pregnancy? The extra lubrication provided by being pregnant can give the vagina a stronger taste or smell which some men notice when giving their wives oral sex. Other than that, there are no medical reasons to stop giving or receiving oral sex during pregnancy unless the pregnancy is at risk for other reasons.

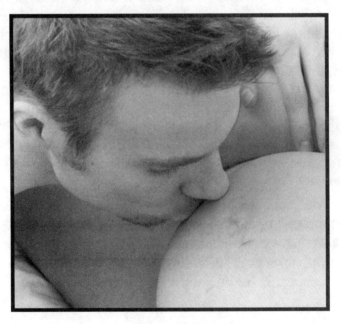

Figure 17: Pregnancy

Very pregnant women find the sideways position the most comfortable. In the sideways position, the female lies on her side. The man can use her thigh as a pillow, lying on his left side, nose to mons, or right side, chin to mons.

Medical Problems That Affect Sexuality

Hysterectomy

It is commonly reported by the medical establishment that if the ovaries are not removed in a hysterectomy, a woman's hormonal cycle and consequently her sexuality are not affected. But what do we actually KNOW about sexuality and a complete hysterectomy, which includes removal of the uterus?

The uterus contracts during sex, so if there is no uterus, there may not be the same sensations of pleasure. Some women report orgasms occurring in the place where the uterus once lay, while other women report enjoying sex less. Sadly, doctors rarely inform women of this possibility before performing a hysterectomy so women are unaware of this downside to surgery.

Other Problems

Other medical problems that may affect a woman's sexuality are endometriosis, interstitial cystitis and fibroid tumors. These can all cause pain during sexual arousal or intercourse.

Medications can also lower a woman's desire, especially antidepressants like Prozac. Of women who take the drug, 13—26% will suffer from an inability to orgasm. Once again, this is usually not something your doctor is going to tell you.

Non-orgasmic

If your partner is unable to have an orgasm, even with oral sex, she may have learned to say no to her sexual feelings. This is especially true if she has little or no experience with childhood or adult masturbation. The desire to be "good" can literally cut off the feelings in our sex organs. Extreme repression can block the pathways of the nervous system that carry genital sensations to the brain.

There is plenty of literature and information available to help a woman learn to be orgasmic. Learning how to masturbate is a great beginning. When a woman masturbates, she learns to like her own genitals and comes to understand what they will and won't do. She learns to enjoy orgasms and becomes proficient in sex. She grows independent of a male partner, which is especially valuable if he is the kind who is uncomfortable with a sexually proficient woman.

Masturbation can make women more at ease and sex more fun. It also makes a woman responsible for her own orgasm. My book, *Five Minutes to Orgasm Every Time You Make Love—Female Orgasm Made Simple*, states:

> Through masturbating yourself, you will learn the difference between the clitoris, labia, urethra, and vagina. Masturbation will help you become more orgasmic and a better sexual partner. It will enable you to assume responsibility for your share of the sex act, more capable of giving and receiving pleasure.

Becoming responsible for one's own orgasm is a basic statement about individuality and equality. Women have a choice when it comes to lovemaking and don't have to depend upon the skills of their lovers. It has less to do with the idea of romance, and more to do with utilitarianism. Thus, it may cause discomfort in the more traditional types, but it brings the physical delights of erotic lovemaking to the forefront.

Some women have little orgasms that occur within moments of contact that are similar to men's early ejaculations. Both sexes can learn to overcome the urge to come too quickly by masturbating.

PC Muscles

The PC muscle is a sling of muscle that supports the sexual organs. They are as much an integral part of orgasm as the clitoris or G-Spot. Well-toned PC muscles can go a long way toward improving orgasms, but chronic tension or weakness can hinder sexual response.

Kegel

Specific exercises originally developed by Dr. Arnold Kegel will improve the tone of these muscles. Kegel initially developed the exercises to help his patients with urinary problems, but a healthy PC muscle also enhances orgasm.

You can isolate this muscle by stopping the flow of urinate in the middle of urination. (Do not make this a regular practice because it may cause a urinary tract infection.) By rhythmically squeezing and releasing the PC muscle, especially with something inside the vagina to work the muscle against, you can produce subtle genital sensations that grow stronger with practice. The movement is the opposite of bearing down as in childbirth—lifting up instead of bearing down. A typical set of exercises would include clenching slowly and then relaxing ten times; clenching as fast as you can ten times and pushing outwardly ten times. Work up to 30 repetitions within each set, several times a day.

Benefits

Benefits other than orgasm include decreasing the likelihood of bladder problems, having an easier time with childbirth and a lessened likelihood of suffering from a prolapsed uterus. Periods may become more regular and a healthy PC muscle can decrease cystitis or vaginal infections.

Maintaining an Erection

Occasionally when a man feels his hard-on starting to go, he will surface from between a woman's legs and try to have intercourse before it is "too late." If he "goes soft," he may not feel as manly. But the kind of concentration needed to maintain an erection is different from the kind needed to perform oral sex. Cunnilingus can be intensely enjoyable for him as well as for you without necessarily making him hard.

You can help keep him hard, however, by performing a few basic tasks. Be sure to tug on your bush to remove any loose hairs, trim your triangle closely and clean the labia at least once a day.

It is important to like your own body and give him more information. If you do not orgasm fast enough, try masturbating yourself while he is giving you oral sex. Above all else, use humor as an important sex aid.

Pain and Cramping

How long will oral sex last? It could be a minute or two or the man could be licking for a long time. Tongue cramping and jaw paralysis are common side effects. They can occur just before the woman blurts out, "don't stop!" "Being able to continue when every ligament and muscle fiber from his neck up is screaming for mercy is what separates the oral sex men from the oral sex boys," says the author of *Guide to Getting it On*.

To combat fatigue, the man should pace himself by keeping a steady, slow, methodical pace. If his neck, arms or tongue begin to ache, he can change positions. He can try using his fingers in place of the tongue for a while.

Men, your fingers are much less sensitive than your tongue, so be careful you are not doing it too hard. Finding a body position that works best for you and your partner in the beginning will go a long way to help you avoid fatigue.

Exercises

Men, if you want to be able to perform for extended periods of time, you can strengthen the muscles in your mouth with exercise. The following are some of the tongue exercises and positions for performing successful cunnilingus:

Exercise 1: Stick your tongue as far out of your mouth as possible, and then try to touch your nose. Holding the rest of the mouth still, begin moving your tongue around clockwise, counterclockwise, and up and down. Repeat in sets of 5.

Exercise 2: Keeping your jaw loose, point your tongue while simultaneously trying to keep your tongue in constant contact with the top and bottom your mouth. Once you are in this position, practice moving your tongue in and out of your mouth.

Exercise 3: Stick your tongue straight out of your mouth, but keep it flat and relaxed. While holding this position, curl the tip of the tongue upward, downward and side-to-side. Practice in five sets.

Exercise 4: With your tongue relaxed and your mouth open, move your tongue in and out of your mouth forward and pull it back. Repeat in sets of five.

Blowing into the Vagina

Should your partner blow into the vagina while performing oral sex? There is a slight chance that an embolism (a gas bubble in the bloodstream, which can be deadly) could happen if a guy were to blow extremely hard into your vagina. However, it would probably take a hard, ceaseless blow into that "sealed" opening to create such an impact. Imagine blowing hard into a balloon with a tiny opening, with your mouth straining. That's the kind of blowing that is required. Heavy breathing doesn't qualify as that kind of action.

Most oral sex on women includes gentle stroking with the tongue, licking and sucking, but not intense blowing. Some men and women report blowing gently into the woman's vulva region as a way to create a pleasant sensation. That's about the only way that sending air onto or into your most private parts usually occurs.

Oral Sex after Ejaculation

What about oral sex after penetration and ejaculation? Some women find it very exciting to share body fluids, and there is certainly nothing to prohibit it except the desires of the partners involved. It can be a terrific turn on to share love fluids and a man may enjoy tasting both flavors. That, in turn, can turn the woman hot and hotter!

13 The Unfun Part: Safe Sex and Sexually Transmitted Diseases

Women's Sexuality

Women Romantic?

We have been taught to think of women as "romantic," while men are programmed to ejaculate into each and every available vagina. We think that women are genetically predetermined to couple with males who will offer the best chance to successfully raise a family—they are, in fact, looking for "relationship material."

Evolutionists who propound these theories are the ones who take them most seriously. They sometimes twist facts to fit their theories, and people who question the process are dismissed as fundamentalist quacks. It's interesting how, with changes in economics and politics, more women catch more ejaculations from more men than they did fifty years ago.

The Pill

Both men and women are having more sex than they did fifty years ago. And contrary to popular thought, Viagra is not the "best friend of the hard penis and wet vagina." The birth control pill holds that distinction. The introduction of the pill enabled women to be more freely passionate and to have as many partners as they wished. The sexual revolution of the 1970s was the beginning. Masters and Johnson published their research on women and sexuality. Then, The Hite Report was the first real statement from women about women's sexuality.

For a period of 10 years or so after the introduction of the birth control pill, people were free to enjoy sex without fear. But early in the 1980s, AIDS and other diseases began appearing and took away the carefree nature of sex.

Oral Sex as Alternative

Oral sex is not a completely safe alternative to vaginal or anal sex. However, unprotected cunnilingus carries a lower risk for transmission of sexually transmitted diseases (STDs) than unprotected vaginal and anal intercourse, or a just-shared, unprotected sex toy, or fellatio. However, there is still some risk for both the giving and receiving partner and some STDs are easier to transmit than others.

Warning Signs of STDs

You probably have an STD if:

1. Your genitals, anus or mouth sprout warts or grow tiny cauliflowers;
2. Lesions or strange looking pimples appear;
3. You experience discomfort when you urinate or your urine is cloudy or has blood in it; and
4. You have a weird discharge or things just don't feel right.

If you experience any of these signs, you should go to a doctor or clinic. Most problems can be treated without pain or hassle. If you do not have the problem looked at by a physician, you could become sterile from a treatable disease. You can also pass sexual infections to your partners without experiencing symptoms yourself.

If you've had more than one sexual relationship during the past year, you should go to a clinic for a checkup. Ask the doctor to include a throat culture if you've been performing oral sex or a rectal culture if you've done anal. Even if you have faithfully used a condom, it is still possible (but not likely) to get some diseases. Also, you can't assume the infection is cured if your symptoms suddenly disappear. Go to a doctor anyway.

AIDS

Spread Through Bodily Fluids

AIDS is a disease or cluster of diseases that involves a shutdown of the immune system. The HIV virus, which is one of the causes of AIDS, is transmitted when the blood of an infected person enters another person's bloodstream through a cut, sore or blood vessel. HIV has also been found in small amounts of semen, vaginal fluid, breast milk and tears. There are several factors that cause it to spread.

AIDS Not Epidemic in North America

There was a time when all we heard was the danger of AIDS spreading into the heterosexual population at the rate it affected the homosexual community. It never, however, made the crossover in North America that was expected. Other sexually transmitted infections have been soaring in straight populations. Why not AIDS? If it were a normal virus, straight college students in the United States would be dying all over the country.

The medical establishment can't explain why few straight people have AIDS when gay men are at high risk. There is a strong association between using recreational drugs and getting AIDS. Few female prostitutes get AIDS as long as they don't use drugs. But there have been very few questions asked of the medical community regarding the current medical predictions. They don't tolerate discussion in the scientific community very well. The same thing happened with hormone therapy. It was thought it should work and so everyone, your local MD included, assumed it would. Until a major study is done, it will be the same with HIV. Then comes the "Oops!" factor.

What about Africa where AIDS is killing millions? Severe malnutrition can result in AIDS symptoms, so it is likely that malnutrition is a greater problem than we realize and AIDS is less of a problem. We might save more lives in Africa by helping to stop malnutrition and by installing water purification systems than by exporting billions of dollars of toxic drugs to treat AIDS.

Transmission through Oral Sex

Transmission of HIV through fellatio or cunnilingus is relatively rare. Unprotected oral sex may put you at risk, however, especially if you have a sore on your lips or in your mouth. But if AIDS were easily transmitted by oral sex, prostitutes would get it in droves. They typically don't get it unless they also shoot up. Still, there is no cure for HIV, and it can be transmitted even when there are no symptoms. Extreme caution is necessary.

Bacterial STDs

There are a number of bacterial sexually transmitted diseases. Trichomonaisis, bacterial vaginosis (BV) and vulviovaginal candidasis (yeast infections) can develop on their own through the growth of harmful bacteria in the vagina. They can be spread through unprotected vaginal intercourse. Trichomonaisis and BV can spread through contact with vaginal secretions, although contracting a yeast infection this way is rare. These diseases can be easily treated with antibiotics.

Gonorrhea, Chlamydia, and syphilis are also bacterial and can be treated with antibiotics. Before 1492, when

Columbus came to America, there had been no recorded cases of syphilis in Europe. It did not exist in the new world, but shortly after Columbus's return, a vicious strain of syphilis spread throughout Europe, quickly killing a large portion of the population. From 1493 until 1550, syphilis was a savage killer. Smallpox got its name because the lesions were small compared to those of The Great Pox syphilis. After 1550, syphilis went from being a quick killer to a slow killer, lingering in the body for years after the initial infection and eventually targeting organs like the heart or brain. It remained a potent killer for 400 years. Half of all hospitals worldwide were filled with its victims.

Syphilis is much less potent today. It is spread through unprotected sexual intercourse. It can also be spread through oral/vaginal contact.

Other STDs

Hepatitis

Hepatitis (plural hepatitides) is characterized by the presence of inflammatory cells in liver tissue. The condition can be self-limiting, healing on its own, or it can progress to liver scarring. The hepatitis viruses cause most of the liver damage worldwide. Hepatitis can also be due to toxins (notably alcohol), other infections or from the autoimmune process. Acute hepatitis lasts six months. It may run a subclinical course when the affected person may not feel ill. Chronic hepatitis is when the disease lasts longer than six months. The patient becomes unwell and symptomatic when the disease impairs liver functions.

Hepatitis A, B and C are viruses that infect millions and can be asymptomatic for years. Hepatitis A is transmitted by oral-fecal contact and an infected partner. Hepatitis B is similar in transmission to HIV. It is found in the blood and other body fluids. You can contract it when fluids from a carrier enter your body via an opening such as a cut or sore. Cunnilingus offers the most risk for Hepatitis B. Hepatitis C is transmitted solely through blood contact. The receptive partner must be menstruating, and the person going down must have a cut, sore or abrasion in their mouth. Hepatitis A is not chronic or long term. There are now vaccines to prevent Hepatitis B, but Hepatitis C has no cure or vaccine.

Herpes and Chlamydia

Chlamydia is a common sexually transmitted disease and a major cause of human eye and genital disease. *Chlamydia trachomatis* is naturally found living only inside human cells and is one of the most common sexually transmitted infections in people worldwide—about 2.8 million cases of Chlamydia infection occur in the United States each year. Chlamydia can cause sterility in women, yet the symptoms are often minimal or non-existent.

Herpes is an extremely contagious STD that is spread through contact with the mucous membranes of an infected person. It can be spread from vulva to mouth and from mouth to vulva, skin to skin, such as using one's hand to stimulate the vulva or anus of the partner. Herpes can be contacted easily when your lover has a cold sore. Even though the herpes virus is benign when it is not active, it is possible to contact Herpes between eruptions (of sores) when the skin is shedding. An outbreak can range from a collection of blistering, painful sores to one small sore that can be unknowingly tucked in a fold of skin. A herpes flare-up will go away on its own. If you are a carrier, however, you need to know so that you don't pass it on to others. If you have sores on the labia, or any discharge, go to the doctor. It is also important to get regular checkups. Many diseases can be treated with antibiotics in their early stages for a complete cure. There is no cure for Herpes. However, treatments in the form of drugs can help prevent the onset of eruptions and decrease the severity of the disease.

HPV

Human papillomavirus is the virus known as genital warts. It is transmitted through skin to skin and mucous membranes when the virus is shedding. There is no cure, but treatments include freezing the warts for removal.

One reason to be especially cautious of this disease is that the virus can cause cancer of the cervix and is also implicated in cancer of the penis.

Mouth Cancer

Oral sex has been linked to a tiny risk of mouth cancer. After a study of 1600 patients with oral cancer from Europe, Canada, Australia, Cuba and the Sudan in 2004, the International Agency for Research on Cancer in Lyon, France found that the patients with oral cancer associated with HPV16 were three times more likely to report having had oral sex than those without the virus strain. HPV16 is the most common strain associated with cervical cancer.

Both cunnilingus and fellatio can infect the mouth, but it is very low risk. The risk is about one person in 10,000 compared to 75-90% of cases that are caused by heavy drinking and smoking. The combination of tobacco smoke and alcohol is thought to produce high levels of cancer causing agents. But oral sex may be the explanation for others who are very young and don't smoke or drink.

Protection

Latex

Because STDs can remain dormant for months or even years, it is possible to transmit something you don't even know you have. That's why barriers are important. When you come in contact with your partner's sexual fluids or if you have an STD, it is essential to use a latex barrier during cunnilingus. Be sure to use a barrier if you or your partner have a bacterial infection such as Chlamydia or vaginosis. Continue this practice until the treatment is completed, especially if you have tiny cuts in your mouth. Small cuts can be caused by something as seemingly harmless as brushing your teeth.

Cunnilingus

Dental Dams

For safety, you can spread a dental dam over her crotch during oral sex. Although a justifiable safety measure, there are some problems associated with this. First, you have no clue what you are licking. Second, there is a texture problem. The tongue drags over the latex, and it is hard to find and keep the appropriate speed. Household plastic wrap is a better barrier because you can see through it, and it doesn't slow the action.

Condoms

Use condoms as a regular habit. Use them on dildos and on penises for vaginal intercourse, anal intercourse, and for oral sex. If your partner objects, discuss alternatives, such as a vaginal condom. A vaginal condom is actually a female condom and is available from any sex store. You may need a little practice to put it on properly.

Gloves

If your hands are clean and free of cuts or abrasions, and you are not using them for heavy penetration, gloves are not absolutely essential. But if you need the added safety, gloves are inexpensive and easy to use. Keep a box by your bed for safety.

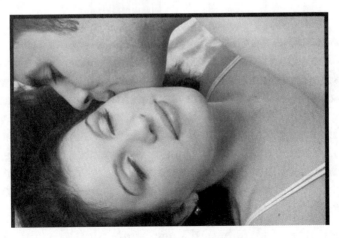

Figure 18: True Intimacy Means Safety

Monogamy

Other than abstinence, monogamy is the ultimate defense against STDs. If both partners have updated tests for STDs and infections and have agreed to have unprotected sex ONLY with each other, you become "fluid bonded."

But don't try to stick with one partner if it is not for you. Never lie to your partner about it. If you can't or won't remain monogamous and don't inform your partner, you may be giving them a death sentence. If either of you take another partner in this arrangement, it is essential to use barriers with other partners, not only to protect yourself, but also to protect your fluid bonded partner. There is nothing worse than infecting an innocent and unknowing partner and, in some instances, it can be treated as a criminal matter.

Don't stop using condoms if there is the slightest chance that you or your partner might have sex outside the relationship. You must be honest and open with each other. Discuss your sexual history with all potential partners. Make an agreement about what kind of precautions you are going to take and stick to them. It is vital to long and short term partnerships in sex not to violate agreements and trust. Don't be stupid. Protect yourself.

Protecting Yourself

There is a strong association between using recreational drugs and getting AIDS. So, rather than focusing on one type of disease, why not try to keep your entire body healthy? First and foremost, this means never do recreational drugs such as poppers (nitrile inhalants) or shoot anything into your veins. Poppers and crystal meth remain extremely popular in the fast lane of the gay sex scene. In fact, crystal meth is so popular that even young guys are taking Viagra to help reverse the effects of "crystal dick," which is meth-related impotence.

Keeping your entire body healthy means staying fit, eating well and avoiding all nonessential drugs. It also means using rubbers if you are having anal sex, whether you are heterosexual or homosexual. And if you aren't true blue and monogamous, it means using rubbers during oral and vaginal intercourse as well. This will help decrease the spread of Chlamydia, syphilis, and perhaps HPV and herpes. It will also help decrease your chances of getting any new diseases.

There would be a significant drop in the number of sexually transmitted infections if people dated for a few weeks or months before they had sex. Perhaps the sex would be better, too.

If for any reason, you feel your partner is being unfaithful, it would be perfectly okay to hire a private detective. If it means saving your own life, any measure is not too drastic. Before it gets to this point, however, run a check on any new person you decide to become intimate with. A routine search using an Internet firm is not that expensive, and it will show you if they have any criminal history, marriages or other shady parts of their life they neglected to tell you about. This sounds very distrusting, but need we repeat that we are talking about your life and health here?

Teenagers and Oral Sex

Abstinence vs. Contraception

Teaching abstinence has been promoted as a way of countering the growing problem of teenage sex. Abstinence education programs teach that abstaining from sex is the only effective or acceptable method to prevent pregnancy or disease. They give no instruction on birth control or safe sex.

Have they worked? Depends on who you ask.

In 1995, there were about 100 pregnancies for every 1,000 teenage women age 15-19, according to the Guttmacher Institute. By 2002, this was down to just over 75 per 1,000. According to researchers from Columbia University and the Guttmacher Institute, 86 percent of the decline is attributable to the use of contraception, while only 14 percent is attributable to abstinence. Abstinence promoters wanted to take the credit, but abstinence has only contributed to a small percentage of the overall decline, and none for teens aged 18-19. For 15-17 year olds, abstinence was responsible for about 23 percent of the decline, according to the study published in the American Journal of Public Health.

All sex education includes the basic principle that a guaranteed way not to get pregnant is not to have sex. So the increase in abstinence, mild as it was, could actually be due to education that promotes contraceptives. The trend of decreasing pregnancy rates might also have nothing to do with education. Cultural shifts could be helping teens to become more responsible in exercising birth control—from contraceptives to abstinence, including oral sex.

Do Abstinence Programs Work?

The impact of abstinence education versus contraception education can be measured by comparing regions within the US that promote abstinence in sex education with regions that primarily teach about contraceptive use. Texas is a leader in abstinence education, but has one of the worst teen pregnancy rates. There could be other reasons other than the type of sex education that Texan teens are getting (like living in a small Texas town, and there's nothing else to do), of course, but there is legitimate evidence that abstinence education is not working. While teen pregnancy rates were going down in Texas, they went down more in other states who did not champion abstinence-based sex education.

Minnesota invested five-million dollars in an abstinence education plan over five years (1998-2002) for certain counties, but not for others. The program was then evaluated. The result? There was no measurable increase in abstinence among young teens (9th graders), but there was a significant decline in sexual activity among 12th graders. Although great news, this could not be explained by abstinence education since 12th graders were too old to participate in it.

After adjusting for a variety of demographic differences

(such as poverty) among different counties, it was found that those counties with no abstinence education funding had *slightly lower* rates of abstinence than those with the abstinence education (49 versus 53 percent). The difference was not significant enough to warrant attribution to the education itself. Any difference in pregnancy rates was not reported. Even Connie Schmitz, the lead author on the study, commented that the program "seems like a really weak intervention," according to the Minneapolis *Star Tribune*.

Abstinence-only education has yielded mixed results. Some of them suggest that abstinence education does delay when teens first have sex, but that when they do, they are less likely to use protection. The Postponing Sexual Involvement (PSI) curriculum (that does not include contraceptive education) showed no positive effects in California.

Does Contraceptive Education Fare Better Than Abstinence Education?

> ... [C]omprehensive sex education includes both information about contraceptives and basic facts about the birds and the bees. It is a simple fact of nature that abstinence is the only 100 percent guaranteed method of birth control. Advocates for Youth found 19 programs it deemed scientifically worthy and which proved their effectiveness in preventing pregnancy, reducing HIV and sexually transmitted diseases, or producing a behavioral benefit such as increased contraceptive use or delaying the onset of sexual activity. Of those that actually decreased pregnancy rates, *all* included contraceptive education.

Contraception v Abstinence Education, Rebecca Goldin, Ph.D., December 12, 2006, www.stats.org

Increase in Oral Sex among Teenagers

Meanwhile, there has been a significant increase in the

proportion of teenagers and young adults engaging in oral sex and, even though much less common, anal sex. The most comprehensive national survey of sexual behaviors ever was released by the federal government. It showed that slightly more than half of American teenagers ages 15 to 19 have engaged in oral sex. Females and males reported similar levels of experience. The prevalence of self-reported oral sex doubled among males (from 16 to 32 percent) and more than doubled among females (14 to 38 percent) from 1994 to 2004. There was also an increase in rectal sex among young women, but it was much less common, rising from 3 percent to 5.5 percent.

Apparently many teenagers have fully accepted the idea that they should not engage in sexual intercourse too soon—intercourse is far too risky. There is a chance of pregnancy and an even greater risk of infection. Teens also consider oral sex more acceptable in their peer group than vaginal sex. The data also underscores the fact that many young people—particularly those from middle- and upper-income white families—simply do not consider oral sex to be as significant as their parents' generation does. They feel that oral sex is far less intimate than intercourse. When 50% of the kids are doing it, that means it is now "normal," an accepted part of teenagers' lives.

As discussed above, even though oral and anal sex prevent pregnancy, they may still result in the transmission of STDs. Young people need to be educated in general about the relative risks for STDs for various sexual behaviors. Parents must be more specific when they discuss sex with their children. If they want their teens to abstain from sex, they need to say exactly what they want their kids to abstain from.

We tend to think that young women who feel the most guilt and shame about sexuality would sleep with fewer guys, but the opposite is true. Girls with the most negative attitudes are doing it younger with more partners and in less committed relationships than girls who feel positive about their bodies and their sexuality. Feeling guilty is more likely to result in first intercourse with an occasional dating partner or with a person they just met and repeating the pattern as they get older. Girls tend to have their first intercourse while drinking or stoned.

Girls who feel better about their bodies tend to masturbate more, but they are not more promiscuous. They tend to wait longer before having first intercourse and have it with more committed partners. High-guilt girls tend to grow up in families where the mother and father are less affectionate toward each other. They regard their dads as over strict and come from homes that are more religious rather than less.

Abstinence programs may prevent intercourse, to a certain extent, but they are not preventing oral and anal sex. Education, not preaching abstinence, is the key to preventing teenage pregnancy and sexually transmitted diseases.

14 Questions and Answers

Aversion to Oral Sex

Question: My boyfriend was raised in a very religious household. He feels that oral sex is too dirty. How can I get him to do it?

Cleanliness issues may involve more than dirt or messiness. A number of people are extremely fastidious, even obsessive, regarding body fluids and avoid any behaviors that lead to their production. Perhaps you can help him examine why he thinks in terms of dirty and clean. Help him consider expanding these definitions in ways that allow greater sharing of sexual freedom.

Unfortunately, many people are just not into performing oral sex for a whole variety of reasons. Some find it too close and personal for their sense of taste or smell. Others have unfounded health concerns and cleanliness issues. Assure them that the vagina naturally cleans itself. Before engaging in any oral lovemaking, be happy to jump into the shower together to

Cunnilingus

ensure that you're both as fresh and naturally fragrant as possible.

People who were raised in very religious homes tend to look down on oral sex. In particular, western religions haven't done well with women and sexuality. Early Christians taught that a virgin daughter occupied a higher place in heaven than her mother since the mother had sex. It was believed that when a boy loses his virginity, he becomes a man. Women, on the other hand, were no longer "pure." In *The Guide to Getting it On*, we learn:

> ... [A]round 400 A.D. St. Jerome wrote, 'Though God can do all things, He cannot raise a virgin after she has fallen' (Epistles 22). Not even God can help you when you lose your virginity, if you are a woman anyway.
>
> Rigid as St. Jerome may have been about women's virginity, he was quite the feminist compared to some of his Christian and Jewish predecessors. For instance, one early church father described women as 'a temple built over a sewer,' with sewer referring to their genitals. Men who made statements like this were later declared saints.

Many adult men and women were raised in households where the temple/sewer notion still exists, and sadly, they will probably never be able to appreciate the beauty of the female body. In order to get past this as a couple, you may need to have an open conversation about the misconceptions of vaginal cleanliness and hygiene. It's important that the man understand that a healthy, clean vagina varies in scent in each woman at different times. It can range from scentless to a slight (or very intense) muskiness. It all depends upon a woman's body, menstrual cycle and current levels of sexual arousal. And while some men find this womanly taste and smell unpleasant or overwhelming, others find it a turn-on.

You can encourage your boyfriend to expand upon his lovemaking experiences with you. Ultimately, however, you will need to respect his choice—if you want to stay together. No one wants to feel coerced into sexual behaviors that are unpleasant to them. If they still do not get into it, let it go and focus on finding other ways for sharing intimate pleasure together. If it is ultimately important to you, you may have to give up on him.

Does Diet Affect Taste?

Question: I am always self-conscious about how I taste down there when my boyfriend is giving me oral sex. He doesn't seem to mind, but I am still concerned. Can what I eat affect the flavor?

Even though it is widely believed that what you eat can affect the smell and taste of your vaginal secretions, there is no scientific research on the subject. Nonetheless, most people believe that what you eat has some effect. You may not always taste great. It depends on how your individual body chemistry reacts with what you eat.

Since your partner loves giving you oral sex, he probably already loves your personal aroma and flavor. But, if you want to play it safe, eat the things that are also good for your overall health. Stick to a diet with lots of vegetables, fruit and whole grains, and try to avoid foods that affect your breath and body odor. A few of these would be garlic, asparagus, spices (like curry) and excess amounts of dairy and animal products.

Helping Him Improve

Question: I need oral sex in order to reach orgasm. Unfortunately, my boyfriend isn't very good at it. What can I say or do that won't hurt his feelings?

The best way to get what you want and have a satisfying

Cunnilingus

sex life is to let your boyfriend know what works for you and what doesn't work for you. Most men appreciate advice. Once they know you're getting off, they get off too. Feel free to ask for what you want. Don't worry about hurting his feelings, but rather than telling him that his oral techniques suck, suggest something like licking you a little faster, or harder, or whatever you may need. You might suggest playing a sex game of follow-the-leader. In follow-the-leader, you go down on him using the kinds of tongue movements you'd like him to use on you. Then, when it's his turn, ask him to use the same techniques on you.

You can also use body language. Push your pelvis toward his mouth or nudge his head in closer if you want more pressure. If you want less pressure, move slightly away from him or gently push his head back a little. If he isn't hitting the right spot, make a V with your index and middle finger and place it around the spot you want him to lick. Other ways to direct him with your fingers are: (1) Pull back the skin on your clitoral hood, which will encourage him to lavish attention on your clitoris, or (2) cover it with your finger if it's too sensitive for direct contact.

It is also important to let him know when he's doing something right. Show, or tell him, when he makes a move that sends you. Give a satisfied moan, and it won't take him long to catch on.

As for requiring oral sex to reach orgasm, there are many books that can teach you how to become orgasmic during intercourse. We'd like to recommend two: *Five Minutes to Orgasm Every Time You Make Love*, by D. Claire Hutchins, and *When the Earth Moves*, by Mikaya Heart. Also check our recommended reading section for more great books.

Asking for Oral Sex

Question: How can I persuade my new boyfriend to go down on me? He loves it when I give him oral sex, but he is not catching the hint to return the favor.

Since oral sex is a very intimate act, you need to make sure that he understands what you are asking for. As long as you ask for what you want in a non-accusatory way, you are not being critical. You are just taking control of your situation. Most guys welcome the feedback and knowing you love it will get him off too.

Next time he's kissing your breasts or belly, tell him in your most sensuous voice, how great it would feel if he went below the belt and kissed you. If he still doesn't get it, he may have a case of performance anxiety. Give him sexy lessons of show and tell. Take his hand and run your tongue along the crease between his thumb and forefinger using the same rhythm and pressure that you'd like him to use on you. Say something like, "This is the way I like to be licked."

If he's squeamish about putting his mouth on your private parts, we've recommended and will always recommend a shower for both of you before you hit the bed. However, if nothing works for him, you will have to decide if a relationship with this man is worth sacrificing your climax. Don't sacrifice yourself and end up regretting it months or years down the road. Remember, there are lots of men who will go down on you without you having to ask. And they will love doing it!

Kissing After Oral Sex

Question: My boyfriend likes to kiss me after he has gone down on me. It makes me a little uncomfortable. Is this normal?

Some couples find it incredibly erotic while others consider the act somewhat taboo. If you have a hygiene issue, you've nothing to worry about, since it's your own body. If you're concerned about the taste, you should try tasting yourself by wetting the tip of your finger in your vagina and tasting it. Personal preference is most important. You need to do what makes you feel comfortable. Perhaps that means not trying it at all and letting your boyfriend know that the idea makes you feel uneasy. Or, you may decide to have that deep kiss in the heat of passion, discovering that it intensifies the intimate bond you two already share.

Sixty-Nine

Question: When we do 69, my boyfriend likes to be on top. I feel like I am choking. How can I be more comfortable?

When your guy is on top during simultaneous oral sex, try pleasing him without taking his entire shaft in your mouth. Lick and kiss the head of his penis, or run your tongue up and down the shaft. He can also hover over you on all fours, his knees by your ears. There are other 69 positions that can be just as mutually satisfying. Why not switch to the woman-on-top pose?

The pleasure plus for you is being able to control the intensity of oral pressure against your clitoris by how hard you press against him. Or, try side-by-side, with your mouths directly in front of each other's genitals. Bend your top legs at the knee and put your feet flat on the mattress. Then you can rest your heads on the lower thigh. It may take some minor modifications before your bodies comfortably mesh, but the beauty of this position is being able to watch the other get off.

Vaginal Farts

Question: Sometimes when my husband performs oral sex and fingers my vagina at the same time, all the air in my vagina comes out and makes a farting noise. It can be very embarrassing, even with my husband.

Occasionally air gets trapped in the vagina and can make a fart-like noise when it comes out. This can happen at any time to any woman and is nothing to be embarrassed about. It is normal room air and unlikely to have any odor. It is most likely to happen when you have had an orgasm. The rear part of the vagina balloons open during arousal and can make a farting noise as it begins to collapse into its normal resting state.

One of the more popular slang expressions for these vaginal "farts" is "keefers."

15 Giving Can Be as Good as Getting

Do men enjoy giving oral sex? And is there a way that you can enjoy giving cunnilingus as much as she enjoys receiving it? Well, almost as much as she enjoys it.

Why would a man deny himself the pleasure of giving oral sex to his partner? Surprisingly, there are some men who just do not enjoy it. Possibly because going down on a woman isn't exactly easy and some guys end up fumbling and feeling embarrassed. And, if she doesn't get off with this ultimate turn-on, is he a complete loser as a lover?

Hang in there. Patience, healthy free-flowing communication and lots of energy will help make oral sex—one of the most beautiful and intimate activities in the world—an easy and enjoyable part of your lovemaking routine. We created this book to enlighten you and we hope you will study it carefully.

Performing cunnilingus masterfully is an important first step. And for some men, the smell, taste and closeness of cunnilingus are their biggest turn-ons. Some guys enjoy being "used" as "sex toys," setting aside their need to be macho for a little while.

One of the principal problems with oral sex is the lack of playfulness. If you approach oral sex under orders, like you have a difficult job to do, it spoils all the fun. Don't let cunnilingus become an "issue." Approach it with a sense of fun and playfulness. Otherwise, instead of being perfect and romantic, it will end up being filled with tension and awkwardness.

Since childhood, we are taught that there is reward in sharing equally and being generous. However, this generosity is eventually downplayed as we learn the value of money. As we grow older and lose our childhood innocence, we grow more selfish and more aware of what we want and how we plan to get it. Sadly, this selfishness is translated to all areas of life, even sexuality. When it comes to oral sex, many would not agree that it is better to give than to receive.

This "balance of oral sex" will create either a surplus of sexual pleasure for one partner or a sexual debt for the other. In a relationship, it is obviously better to seek equality, but only to a point. Keeping tally on whose turn is it really will only cause intimacy to seem more like a chore—this week you lick the penis and next week I'll rub the clitoris.

Instead, consider oral sex a pleasure, regardless of role. Do not allow yourself to feel forced into giving oral sex and do not expect to receive every time. By focusing more on the act of oral sex, you can become better at pleasuring your partner. When a couple is focused on each other, oral sex can be an intimate experience shared equally.

Dirty is fun. I don't mean dirty as in unclean. I mean sexy, dirty fun. An important part of the sexual experience is to see the pleasure on her face and the thrill when she pushes her self involuntarily against your face. It will enhance your sexual delight.

When a woman lets go completely, it's a fantastic experience for you both. There's a lot more to oral sex than orgasm. It's about making your lover feel good all over.

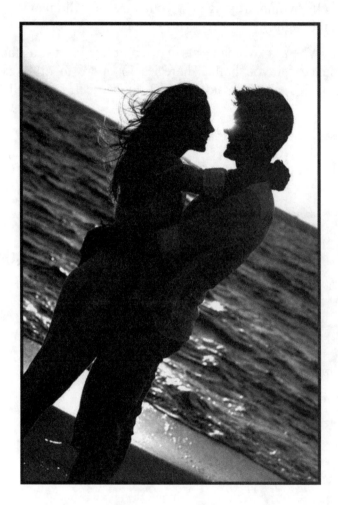

Figure 19: Enjoying Each Other

16 The Emotional Needs of Women

After all is said and done, the act of oral sex belongs to the female clitoris. Even though the clitoris is not the only participant in receiving oral sex, it is by far the star.

Early History

Before the 1960s, few knew what the clitoris was, much less what to call it. That's when the word "clitoris" came into common usage. Many men and women were ignorant of its function. Early sex manuals described it as a "mini-penis," and consequently, men trying to please their partners would rub the clitoris with the intensity they wanted used on their penises. This, of course, didn't work too well and resulted in extreme discomfort for their partners.

The birth control pill came into common usage in the 1960s and became the best friend to sex ever invented. Everything began to change for women with the introduction of the birth control pill.

Getting to that point was rather difficult. When

researchers wanted money to work on the birth control pill, drug companies refused because such an idea was disgusting to them. Being associated with birth control was looked down upon. Goodyear Rubber, which produced $150 million worth of condoms in 1958, refused to acknowledge it. Even as late as 1953, it was still against the law for scientists in Massachusetts to do studies or research on contraceptives.

When first developed, it took the ovaries of 80,000 pigs to extract a tiny bit of estrogen. In order to harvest enough hormones to fit on the head of a pin or two, German biochemists had to collect and distill 25,000 liters or urine from the horses in the police barracks in Berlin. It was a huge leap when researchers learned to synthesize the hormones needed for birth control pills from yams grown in Mexico. And contrary to what is believed today, most women who lined up to get the first birth control pills were not single, but mothers in their 30s and 40s with three to six children. They lined up at doctor's offices the moment it became available.

Why Women Love

When you give a woman oral sex, she feels like more than just a sex partner. She feels more loved than when she's treated as a cook or your housekeeper or babysitter to your children. Learning to give the best oral sex you possibly can requires understanding a woman's anatomy and what gives her the most pleasure. In addition, it requires trust, lust and communication between both partners. Even if it is a one night stand or a ten year relationship, with a little dose of horniness, the possibilities for oral fulfillment with your partner are endless. Whether you remain simple friends or become true partners for life, performing cunnilingus can be one of the most wonderful things you can do for a woman. It makes her feel loved, admired and sexy.

Many women prefer oral sex to intercourse and, for those who require a large amount of clitoral stimulation, it is the easiest way to orgasm. Many women expect it these days.

Men who perform great cunnilingus are always

Cunnilingus

appreciated and considered fabulous lovers. The act of cunnilingus should be approached openly and without doubt. It is impossible to intellectually learn how to love your partner, and it can't be faked. If you don't enjoy it and are reluctant to perform oral sex, it will show. Oral sex proves to her that you fully accept her as a sexual being and that you love every intimate part of her. There is no place on her body that you consider dirty or off limits.

Sharing sex with a partner allows you to discover different emotions, hopes and dreams, laugher and pain and what it takes to free the fun, passion, and hidden kinkiness in your lover's body. To achieve that level, you have to take the time to know someone, to feel what they are feeling, to see the world through their eyes, and to let a partner discover who you are in ways that might leave you both feeling vulnerable.

And, lest we forget, oral sex has the potential to give her an exceptional orgasm. It can be fast or it can be a relaxing and healing orgasm. Cunnilingus can take both you and your female partner to new heights of pleasure. Smile, touch her lightly, hold her, tell her how beautiful she is and how good she makes you feel. Your enthusiasm goes further than the best of techniques. Enjoy now and forever!

Index

INDEX

A

AIDS 89, 90, 91, 96
anilingus45, 55, 64, 66, 67, 68, 69, 70
Aromatherapy 27
autocunnilingus 58

B

Basic Instinct 7, 54
Beaver 21
Bert Herrman 44
birth control pill 11, 89, 113, 114
Bondage 71, 75
Buzzing .... *See* Hummer

C

cancer
  oral 94
cavernosal artery 9
clitoral hood 9, 22, 33, 35, 38, 105
Coming Home 59
condom
  vaginal 95
corpora cavernosa 9
cortisone 23
crura 9

D

dental dam 68, 95
dildo 70, 77

Durex 50

E

E. coli 66, 67
ejaculation
  female 61

F

Face Sitting 57
fellatio 2, 15, 17, 44, 49, 89, 91, 94
finger cots 68
Fisting 43

G

Gene Simmons 1
glycerin 20
Good Will Hunting 54
G-spot 43, 60, 61
Guttmacher Institute 97

H

Henry and June 54
hepatitis 66, 92
herpes 66, 93, 97
Hite Report 89
HIV 66, 67, 90, 91, 92, 99
hummer 45, 57

J

Jane Fonda 59
Jehovah's Witnesses 79
Jon Voight 59

K

Kama Sutra 2, 17, 54
keefers 108
Kegel 85

L

labia ... 7, 8, 16, 18, 21, 22, 23, 24, 29, 30, 31, 32, 36, 37, 38, 40, 45, 58, 84, 85, 93
lactobacilli 18, 19
lubrication 36, 65, 82

M

massage
    erotic 27
    genital 29
Masters and Johnson 12, 89
menstruation 81
mons veneris ..... 38, *See* pubic mound
mucous membrane 36

N

Nancy Friday 30

O

orgasm
    disappearing 40
orgasms
    clitoral 12
oxytocin 27

P

PC muscles 84
perineum 8
periurethral sponge .... See G-spot
phone sex 74
pill
    birth control 89
position

classic 55
doggie 56, 69
kneeling 56
sixty-eight 45
sixty-nine .... *See*
Prozac 83
pubic mound 7, 29, 31

R

revolution
    sexual 12, 72, 89
Rimming .... See anilingus

S

Sadism/Masochism 75
saliva 20, 32, 36, 45, 57, 65
scrotum 8
Secret Garden 30
sexually transmitted diseases .. 89, 91, 93, 94, 99, 101
shame 16, 17, 50, 53, 100
Sharon Stone 7
South Pacific Trobriand Islanders .. 62
Squirting 61, 63
STDs .... *See* sexually transmitted diseases
Stiff Upper Lips 54

T

Taoism 2
The Hand Book 44
tipping the velvet 3

U

urinary canal 61

V

vagina .. 2, 7, 9, 13, 14, 18, 19, 20, 22, 32, 37, 38, 42, 43, 46, 52, 60, 61, 65, 66, 68, 78, 82, 84, 85, 87, 88, 89, 91, 102, 103, 106, 107
vaginal secretions 19, 91, 104
vestibular bulbs 9
vestibular glands 8
vibrator 42, 43, 45, 46, 57, 61, 75, 77, 78

vulva 8, 10, 18, 20, 22, 29, 31, 35, 36, 37, 42, 46, 61, 68, 69, 75, 87, 93

W

warts 66, 89, 93
wax
    Brazilian 24

waxing
    genital area 23
When the Earth Moves 105

Y

yoni kisses 2

Bibliography & Glossary

<u>Was that an earthquake?</u>

The Sensuous Couple's Guide to Seismic Oral Sex

D. Claire Hutchins
Avery Sinclair

JPS Publishing Company
Dallas, Texas

Was that an earthquake?
The Sensuous Couple's Guide to Seismic Oral Sex
By
D. Claire Hutchins
Avery Sinclair

Published by: JPS Publishing Company, Dallas, Texas
www.jpspublishing.com

All rights reserved. No part of this book may be reproduced or transmitted in any form or by any means, electronic or mechanical, including photocopying, recording or by any information storage and retrieval system without written permission from the publisher, except for the inclusion of brief quotations in a review.

Copyright © 2008 by D. Claire Hutchins and Avery Sinclair

Publisher's Cataloging-in-Publication
(Provided by Quality Books, Inc.)

Hutchins, D. Claire.
 Was that an earthquake? : the sensuous couple's guide to seismic oral sex / D. Claire Hutchins, Avery Sinclair.
 p. cm.
 Includes bibliographical references and index.
 LCCN 2008923254
 ISBN-13: 978-0-9664924-5-3
 ISBN-10: 0-9664924-5-5

 1. Oral sex. 2. Sex instruction. I. Sinclair, Avery. II. Title. III. Title: Sensuous couple's guide to seismic oral sex.

HQ31.5.O73H88 2008   613.9'6
                            QBI08-600091

BOOK TWO

Fellatio

Avery Sinclair

Disclaimer

This book provides information regarding the covered subject matter. Neither the publisher nor the authors is engaged in rendering legal, medical, accounting, psychiatric or psychological, or other professional advice. If expert assistance is needed, the services of a professional should be sought.

This book does not contain all the information that is available on this subject. For more information, see the references in the Bibliography section.

The sole purpose of this book is to entertain. The authors and the publisher have no liability or responsibility to any person or entity with respect to any loss or damage caused, or alleged to be caused, directly or indirectly, by the information in this book.

Table of Contents
Book Two - Fellatio

ILLUSTRATIONS

1 IS IT WORK OR IS IT FUN?.......................... 1
    How We Feel About It..1
    Common Goals 4

2 WHOSE IDEA WAS THIS? 7
    History 7
    Why Men Want It 11
    Why Women Want to Do It 12
    The Gay Perspective 13

3 CAN SETTING THE MOOD MAKE IT BETTER?... 15
    Foreplay..15
    Fantasy 17

4 HOW IT WORKS: THE ANATOMY OF MALE SEXUAL AROUSAL 21
    The Outer Body..22
    What Goes on Inside? 25

5 SPECIAL SPOTS AND SPECIAL ISSUES .. 31
    Sweet Spot 31
    Prostate..31
    Anus 32
    What Special Issues Arise (No Pun Intended)? ...32
    Sight 32
    Sound 34
    Smell 34
    Taste...35
    To Swallow or Not to Swallow..............................37
    Emotional Needs of Men 38

6 GETTING STARTED 39
    Psychology...39

	Cleanliness..*43*
	Communication...*48*
	Experimentation..*49*
7	**TECHNIQUE – MAKE IT SEISMIC!** **51**
	General..*51*
	Hands..*53*
	Mouth..*55*
	Tongue..*56*
	Anus and Internal...*60*
	Premature Ejaculation..*62*
	Orgasm and Ejaculation...*63*
8	**FOR THE ADVENTUROUS – ADVANCED TECHNIQUES**... **65**
	Fellatio in Our Everyday Sex Lives...........................*65*
	Self-Pleasing..*65*
	Advanced Techniques...*68*
9	**SHAKE THINGS UP! NEW POSITIONS**...... **75**
	Versatility...*75*
	Positions...*75*
10	**FANTASIES AND PRACTICES**.................... **83**
	Fantasies...*83*
	Practices...*84*
11	**DEVICES AND TOYS**....................................... **87**
	Pain as Pleasure..*87*
	Pleasure without Pain..*90*
12	**BELIEVE IT OR NOT**....................................... **99**
	Facts...*99*
	Myths of Male Sexuality...*100*
	Problems...*101*
13	**SAFE ORAL SEX**... **105**
	Risks of Unprotected Fellatio...................................*106*
	Warnings and Suggestions..*106*
	Condoms and Other Protections................................*108*

14	**COMMON & UNCOMMON QUESTIONS**	**113**
15	**THE EMOTIONAL NEEDS OF MEN**	**117**
	Over-Simplification of Male Sexuality	*117*

INDEX 119

GLOSSARY AND BIBLIOGRAPHY 123

Illustrations credits

Original artwork by Sed Kaya, Sed Kaya Productions, Winter Garden, Florida

Historical and other drawings in Public Domain

Cover by Juanita Dix, Florida

The Authors

Avery Sinclair and D. Claire Hutchins are teachers and sex educators who reside in the suburbs of Dallas, Texas.

ILLUSTRATIONS

Figure 1: Édouard-Henri Avril .... Frontpiece
Figure 2: Iris reanimates deceased Osiris 8
Figure 3: Feel Free to Fantasize 18
Figure 4: Circumcised Penis, Erect and Unerect 22
Figure 5: Penis Circumcised and Uncircumcised 26
Figure 6: Male Reproductive System 29
Figure 7: The Star 34
Figure 8: The First Time 40
Figure 9: Condom 49
Figure 10: Basic Technique 52
Figure 11: Using the Hand 55
Figure 12: Rimming 61
Figure 13: Deep Throat 70
Figure 14: The Principal Position 78
Figure 15: Seated Position 79
Figure 16: Félicien Rops Engraving 82
Figure 17: Butt Plug 90
Figure 18: Fun Furry Handcuffs 91
Figure 19: Strap-on 92
Figure 20: Manual Installation 109
Figure 21: Putting a Condom on With Your Mouth 110
Figure 22: Men Have Emotional Needs too 116

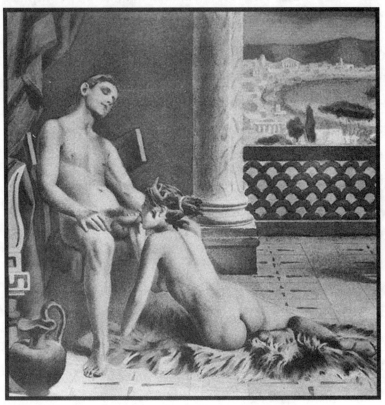

Figure 1: Édouard-Henri Avril
1843-1928

1 Is It Work or Is It Fun?

How We Feel About It

What is Fellatio?

"Fellatio" is defined as the placing of one human being's mouth onto the penis of another human being with carnal intent. For a heterosexual, this means the female mouth on a male penis. It can also mean male-on-male, or, in the extreme, a man's mouth on his own penis (called "auto-fellatio").

Regardless of whomever is doing it to whomever, the visualization of fellatio conjures up grainy porno movies. We imagine sleazy crash pads with orange shag carpeting, and a skanky looking female going down on a balding man still wearing his socks. These images, gleaned mostly from movies made during the seventies, make fellatio look dirty. Many people still feel this way, even in our more liberated times.

Regardless of how we feel about fellatio, or think we should feel, the truth is that it is a fairly universal practice. The American love/hate relationship with fellatio may be a hangover from our Puritan roots. It still remains an act that can bring a great deal of pleasure to both participants. In actuality, there is nothing inherently bad or good about fellatio. It is merely a sexual activity.

What sets fellatio apart from other sexual acts is its intimacy. One person comes face-to-face with the most private part of a man's body. The genitals are even referred to as "private parts." The anticipation of such proximity and strangeness—having our noses in another person's most intimate space—can produce huge fears. Are we going to be able to perform our task properly? We want to give our man the greatest pleasure that we are able to, but are our efforts going to be rewarded by his happiness? And the biggest fear of all—are we going to look ridiculous?

The purpose of this book is to quell those fears. We intend to give you enough information, suggestions and practices that you will feel perfectly comfortable giving your significant other the ultimate pleasure. You will, in fact, look forward to it. Every encounter with his member will be a pleasurable and rewarding experience for you both.

Versatility

One of the major advantages of fellatio is its versatility. It can be performed almost anywhere and at any time you feel like it. The front seat of an automobile, for example, is a highly inconvenient place for intercourse (doable, but awkward). But giving your guy a blowjob from the passenger seat is a cinch, and something he will very much appreciate. One precaution, however. Do not try this in a MOVING vehicle, especially after you have read this book. He will be so into what you are doing that he may completely lose his concentration. We wouldn't want to be responsible for serious injuries. Perhaps the authorities should make the same law for fellatio that they do for cell phones: *no blowjobs in school zones!*

Seize a few moments of privacy whenever you can, and perform this highly adaptable sex act. What about a semi-public

Fellatio

place? The anticipation of getting caught can heighten the excitement. Maybe a children's slide in a city park (late at night only, when there's no chance of any little children happening by)? It isn't worth getting arrested or causing an old lady to have a heart attack. So be careful where you decide to play. Even the privacy of your own bedroom could be an exciting place to perform fellatio.

Fellatio is adaptable in other ways as well. You may have a way of doing it that is exclusive to you. Or, if you are the receiver, you may have personal preferences that the giver could easily accommodate. It all depends on who is giving and who is receiving, and their knowledge of techniques, toys and choices. The positions and styles are endless and are enough for any lifestyle, personal choice or situation. It is so accommodating that you may even be able to come up with some variations of your own. Perhaps you have decided to indulge in a place most wouldn't think of. Perhaps you would be willing to put some time into it that the average person wouldn't. You may have a partner whose personal choices are different, but you are ready and willing to accommodate them. Have fun with it!

Another way that fellatio demonstrates its versatility is with men who have disabilities. For example, back trouble and paralysis lend themselves well to being accommodated by fellatio. If the other party is unable to participate at all, the giver can do it on inanimate objects, like a strap-on or a vegetable. The same technique can be used to revitalize a languid sexual relationship as it will stimulate the senses. You might want to learn to perform "deep throat." This technique is not for everyone, as it takes some time, dedication and practice to learn. If you do learn it, you will drive your partner mad with ecstasy.

Few things limit fellatio beyond the minds, spirits and willingness of its participants.

Common Goals

Overcoming Fears

Both parties participating in the love act of fellatio can have many fears. For example, the man who is receiving the procedure could be worrying about his penis. In no other act will his member be so close to his beloved. It appears in Technicolor, bigger-than-life, with all its warts, crooks and crannies, smells and feelings. He probably thinks it's too small. You're probably glad! He might think it is shaped funny. You might need a good laugh. He might be afraid he won't be able to get it up. You're probably afraid he won't be able to get it off, and you will be doing this the rest of the night. He may have latent sexual shame from his mommy swatting his hand every time he played with his baby winky. Your sexual shame is greater, because you're about to put that thing in your mouth!

If it is your first time, or if you have had prior bad experiences, you might not like giving fellatio. The sight of a turgid penis might send you screaming into a dark corner. You may curl into a fetal position that would put Emily Rose to shame. Maybe his weenie looks like a sap—those rubber things police officers use to club unruly criminals. Maybe it feels like a slimy frog. What if it tastes that way, too?

You fear you wouldn't know what to do with it even if you did manage to get it past your lips. He'll think you look ridiculous with his penis in your mouth. You think you'll look like my dog. She takes her cigar-shaped chewy treats into her mouth lengthwise rather than horizontally. It looks like she's smoking a cigar. Your man will laugh when he sees you smoking his cigar. By now, you are so mortified and carried-away with your crazy thoughts, you don't want to come anywhere near his penis.

Lighten up! These fears and misgivings can be dealt with in numerous ways. Begin by having a common goal when it comes to fellatio.

Fellatio

Having Fun

If you don't already have one, acquire a sense of humor. Humor is the best way to overcome fear. Always try to keep in mind that the other person feels as awkward and uncomfortable as you do. Get out of yourself. Concentrate on them rather than you. Your nervousness will be alleviated proportionately.

Don't keep it to yourself. Communicate with your lover, and share some of your misgivings with him. If you do, he will most likely be willing to share some of his. You can both laugh at your own and each other's fears.

Gift of Fellatio

Your man may have been fantasizing about receiving head since childhood. The fact that you willingly give it to him will stimulate his libido immeasurably. While men appreciate vaginal sex, and it is a powerful way of expressing affection, fellatio is the ultimate gift you can give him. It shows him how much you are into him and how much you want to please him. Be assured, he will be pleased. By pleasing him, you will be empowering yourself.

2 Whose idea was this?

History

Masturbation

Men have been entranced with their genitalia from the beginning of time. As diligently as they have sought to satisfy themselves, society has just as diligently been trying to curb their enthusiasm for pleasuring themselves. Doctors, as late as the 20th Century, were warning parents that their sons could develop all manner of conditions if they were allowed to masturbate. Your son, the physicians cautioned, could break out in chronic acne, have seizures or, woe-of-woes, go blind! What were their recommendations for preventing these boys from self-abuse? Spiked cockrings, ice water enemas, erection alarms and circumcision. These prevention methods sound like some of the devises and methods used in the sex toys and techniques sections of this book. These devices, meant to prevent boys from masturbating, merely exposed them to a wider variety of pleasures than they could have imagined by themselves.

Fellatio

Touching his own penis is divine, but having someone else touch it—explosive. When the other person is touching and sucking with their mouth—out of this world! Has this technique been around for a long time, or is it relatively new? Is it only practiced in certain societies or is it universal?

Ancient Societies. Egypt is the first place that traceable evidence of fellatio has been found. It arises from the myth of Osiris and Iris. Osiris was killed by his brother. The brother added insult to injury by cutting Osiris into pieces. Their sister, Iris, tried to put the pieces back together. She was successful up to a point.

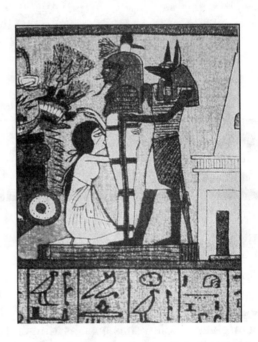

Figure 2: Iris reanimates deceased Osiris

Unfortunately, Osiris' penis was missing. Since the brother wasn't telling where it was, Iris made a penis out of clay. She placed it at the proper place on the body. She "blew" life back into the penis by sucking it, as the myth goes. This is the first record of a woman performing fellatio on a man's penis. Unfortunately, he wasn't alive to enjoy it. Talk about a man's penis having a life of its own! There are still-existing explicit images of this myth.

China of old was like India. Sexually speaking, the society placed very few, if any, taboos or denouncements on the people.

Fellatio

A chapter in the Kama Sutra is devoted entirely to "auparishtaka." The interpretation of this term is "oral congress," which included eight ways of performing fellatio.

The act of fellatio in ancient Rome was described as the opposites of "active" and "passive." The person receiving the fellatio, usually a soldier or virile male, was considered the active participant. The person giving the fellatio, normally a slave or a woman, was considered the passive participant. Today, it is considered just the opposite (by most people). The giver is the active one while the receiver is the passive one.

The Roman concept of active and passive still lingers, primarily in vanishing cultures. In New Guinea, for example, young people are required to practice fellatio on adults as an initiation ritual. This culture holds that sperm is a vital resource. Ingesting it produces strong, macho males. These are not homosexual communities. They are societies in which females are raised to be totally submissive and dominated by males. Happily, as noted above, these cultures are rapidly disappearing.

Fellatio and Religion. According to the Catholic Church, up until the 19th century at least, any sexual activity that did not lead directly to procreation was a sin. Fellatio is still frowned upon by them and many other religious organizations, whether within marriage or without. During the 19th century, when a man and a woman committed a sexual act outside of coitus, they were considered to be practicing "onanism." Dire and dark things would happen to those who insisted on participating in onanism. Men are not supposed to "spill their seed" onto the ground, which Christian groups interpreted as a warning against masturbation and fellatio. Coming in the mouth is not mentioned.

In the condemnation of fellatio, the religion of Islam is in agreement with Judeo-Christians. Their objections are the same: if it does not lead directly to procreation, it should not be practiced. Traditional Islamic cultures, such as black African cultures, associate a taboo with the mouth, which they consider a pure organ. The spoken word of truth comes from the mouth. Since fellatio sexualizes the mouth, it is considered dirty and defiles the mouth. By association, a woman who performs fellatio is dirty—where have we heard that one before?

By the same token, the Inuit culture believes that fellatio takes away their strength. They do not engage in the act at all. Since they kiss with their noses, they do not consider the mouth a sexual object. Consequently, fellatio is taboo.

Fellatio in America. Fellatio rose to the forefront during the seventies. At that time, contrary to the present century, blowjobs were something you did last, after you had participated in real intercourse. It was not something you did instead of intercourse, like teenagers do today. Those days were euphoric because the only real sexually transmitted diseases were syphilis, gonorrhea, warts and crabs. Syphilis and gonorrhea were practically obliterated by the invention of penicillin. Warts and crabs were easily treatable.

It was the birth of women's liberation as well. We had the right to abortion and the pill. It seems that the more intelligent and educated a woman was, the more inclined she was to participate and initiate fellatio. Note that the cultures that discourage education in women also discourage fellatio. No wonder they don't want their women educated. It obviously leads to the performance of fellatio, and consequently, sin.

Perhaps the biggest contribution the 20th century made to the promotion of fellatio was the release of the movie *Deep Throat* starring Linda Lovelace. More blowjobs can be attributed to that particular cultural phenomenon than just about any other.

The second big influence on American attitudes toward fellatio was the President Bill Clinton/Monica Lewinsky scandal. She performed the most famous blow job in the history of the human race. From that time on, teen sex made the move from intercourse to "body part sex." Giving fellatio is deemed to be quick, easy and noncommittal. Every teen male can say he "did not have sexual relations with that woman," simply because he did not engage in intercourse. He was merely on the receiving end of a quickie blowjob.

About 15 states in the US have criminalized fellatio. Ironic, given the fact that the United States of America is by far the biggest producer of pornography on earth. This is strange behavior for a so-called Puritan country. Although pornographic movies are big business in the US, there is very little of it going on in Europe. The vast quantities we produce almost invariably feature fellatio.

Humans Versus Other Species. Human beings are constantly trying to set themselves apart from all other animal species. We are more intelligent; we are mightier; we are able to contemplate our own existence; we fear the unknown of death. What is the single most important event that sets us apart from the other animals? We are forced to wipe after we eliminate. Have you ever seen those baboons with the big rear ends grab a sheet of toilet paper and wipe them off? There is one thing, however, that may truly set us apart from all other animals: humans may be the only animals who give blow jobs.

There is a species of chimpanzees (males) who lick their female mates. That is not fellatio. It is cunnilingus. The act appears to be primarily for the sake of hygiene, or to tempt the female into playing. It does not appear to be a sexual maneuver by the male to give the female an orgasm or to prepare her for intercourse. It is not an act unto itself, but merely a preliminary to other activities. Although it can be used as preliminary activity to other sexual acts, fellatio is basically a sexual act unto itself. In that respect, human beings are where we have always wanted to be—unique in the animal world.

Why Men Want It

Depends on the Man

Men desire fellatio for varying reasons. Some men feel that it puts them into a position of power. They are receiving a service and deriving pleasure from it. Other men prize fellatio above all sexual acts, even intercourse, because it requires complete devotion from their partner. Even though the inside of the mouth and the use of the tongue may mimic the vagina, for men it is different. There are pleasures created by being in someone's mouth that cannot be created by the vagina.

The visual stimulation alone, of seeing his partner's mouth moving up and down on his most prized member, would almost be enough. Combine that with the other physical and mental stimulations that a blow-job provides, and you will have your man worshipping you.

As we all know, there are countless other ways to stimulate a man—hands, breasts, butts, vagina, even sex toys. The glory of fellatio is that it pulls all of these elements together for an ending so incredible that a man will never forget it. **For him, there is no other feeling as powerful as the focused orgasm following fellatio. If he had to choose his last sex act on earth, before he died, he would choose fellatio and die a happy man.**

Why Women Want to Do It

Nice Girls Do it Too

The sights, the sounds, the joy of giving her partner pleasure can turn some women up to high velocity. Often, however, they may experience guilt for feeling this way. They may believe that it is not normal. For the most part, especially among older women, the mere mention of fellatio brings about a universal outcry of disgust. Younger women (twenties and thirties) may be more tolerant, as they are the ones who were giving it to their boyfriends during high school rather than having intercourse. Women who are older were doing their best to put off intercourse until they were either married, in love or "emotionally ready." They would never have considered substituting fellatio for sex, however, even if it does seem rather efficacious. Also, post-menopausal women's reduction in

Fellatio

certain hormones has conversely reduced their sexual desire. This is normal unless they have lost all desire whatsoever.

Regardless of one's age, social position or upbringing, the truth is that liking to give blowjobs is neither abnormal nor shameful. Nice girls absolutely do enjoy sex. They love making their men happy. Don't let anyone try to convince you otherwise.

We may call it a "blowjob," but the truth is, it should be fun, not hard work.

How Do We Get Comfortable with It?

Let's assume you are one of those women for whom the idea of fellatio is off-putting. By writing this book, we are trying to give the "pitcher" (the one who is on the giving end of the blowjob) enough knowledge to give her (or him, if you are gay) enough knowledge in order to become comfortable with fellatio. The catchword is "communication." You must be able to talk with your partner about the act you are about to perform.

Always begin slowly, moving along at your own pace. At first, only try the things that you feel comfortable with. Practice new techniques as you progress. Foremost, and most importantly, have fun with it! This book will present many different techniques and positions. Some may work well for you, others won't. Same for him. The key is to have options and the freedom to choose. It doesn't matter how you get there. The end result will always be great. Once you have discovered the course of your journey, take the same route time and again. When you get tired of that, try something else.

The Gay Perspective

Homosexual vs. Heterosexual

Despite what your feelings may be regarding homosexuality, the fact of life is that men do have sex with other men. Since they do not have vaginas, it is obvious that the most common way men have sex with each other is fellatio.

When it comes to sex, we cannot put people into heterosexual, homosexual, transsexual, or any other kind of box. If you think only gay men suck cocks, then refer to the section on "autofellatio." It answers the question, if you could go down on yourself, would you? And, if you could, would you come in your own mouth?

Even though this book is being written from the female perspective, that is, a female going down on a male partner, anything that is included in this book is also usable for two male partners. This is a book about fellatio. If it is useful to anyone, that is okay with the authors. Some of the other things we will be discussing may be controversial. For example, anal penetration, sex toys and the use of pain to achieve pleasure. If these types of things are not helpful for you, skip those chapters.

The Goal of the Book

The goal of this book is to give the reader all the information they will need in order to perform the act of fellatio with power, knowledge, safety and joy. In order to succeed with that, we must assume our readers are from all areas of sexual orientation.

Fellatio is merely a sex act. It does not have a political, social or religious orientation. Regarding fellatio, neither do we.

3 Can Setting the Mood Make it Better?

Foreplay

Time for Sex

Is it necessary to make time for sex? There is something to be said for the quickie, whether it is fellatio or intercourse. You don't have to plan ahead, it doesn't take long, and you can do it just about anywhere (anywhere, that is, that you are sure of not getting caught). Often, however, making the effort to set aside a prescribed amount of time to make love to your partner can be your best bet. If you have enough time, you can engage in extended foreplay that will make the final orgasm a blockbuster rather than just the old routine.

Pre-Foreplay

Foreplay is not just the physical things you do to each others' bodies a few minutes before the main event. If you have set aside time for sex, it can begin the moment you pop out of bed in the morning. Try giving him a preview of what is to come that evening. Be creative. Give him a peck on his pecker before you jump up to shower before work. Both he and his alter ego will be surprised and delighted. Remind him that it is just the beginning, the first on a list of a great many things that are going to happen to him today. As you begin to dress in front of him, show him a little skin. He won't be able to keep from thinking about you the rest of the day.

Call, email or text message him a few times during the day, giving him subtle hints of the glories that await. Rush home in order to get there before he arrives. Turn off the phone, the TV and the computer. Turn on some music. Make it something sensuous and exciting. Use the dimmer switch on the electric lights, and light some fragrant candles (gardenia is nice). Then it is time for a hot bath with lightly perfumed bath oil and bubbles. Luxuriate for awhile, until you are languorous and feeling sensual. You've heard all this before. You know what to do. By the time he arrives you are relaxed and ready.

Erotic Massage

There are techniques you can learn that will put him into a state of euphoria before you even begin to address his penis. There is no activity that gives a greater overall feeling of pleasure than massage. A regular massage works the muscles beneath the skin while erotic massage primarily works the skin. For some helpful hints, refer to the cunnilingus section of this book. Check the ***Bibliography*** if you want more information.

Before the Sex Act

Now that you have him ozoned out, spend the next few minutes kissing and nibbling everywhere but his genital area. Begin at the top of his head and end with his toes (if you are so inclined). Touch, kiss, nibble and lick every nook and cranny you come across. Be sure to pay special attention to his reactions to these attentions. This is a great way to learn where his erogenous areas are located.

Talking

Have you ever been turned on just by the sound of someone's voice? Most likely, the sound of your voice is erotic music in his ears. Think about a movie where the characters are in total darkness, and all you can hear are the sounds they are making. You would know they were making love just by the sounds coming from the screen. Use your voice to add to his pleasure and anticipation. Make moaning, kissing and licking noises. Say sexy words you believe will heighten his excitement. Some men love to hear you talk dirty. Others may prefer daintier chatter. All men will love one word, the hottest word in the English (or any other) language: his name! Be sure to repeat it at every opportunity. More importantly, be sure you are using the correct name! It is not sexually stimulating to him when you call Thomas by Dexter's name.

Fantasy

Fantasies Make Anything Possible

What is the best thing about having erotic fantasies? That you can have illicit sex with Josh Holloway without your husband's or boyfriend's knowledge? That you can have illicit sex with Josh Holloway, and he won't care if your thighs are flabby? All of the above, of course, and more.

What about fellatio and fantasies? Fellatio lends itself well to fantasy because of its ease of use. It is easy to conjure up a movie star, drop to your knees behind a studio backdrop, and give a fantastic blowjob, or perform any other sex act your libido conjures up. Use this fantasy to make giving your husband of 20 years an amazing blowjob that will be even more exciting for you than it was for him. Believe me, he will notice and respond to your enthusiasm. He won't know you are thinking of a hunky actor instead of him. If he did, he probably wouldn't care anyway.

Maybe you think your boss is hot. Maybe going down on him gives you some power over him that you do not have at the office. You may blush when you see him on Monday morning, but he will never know you used him in an erotic fantasy. What harm could it do?

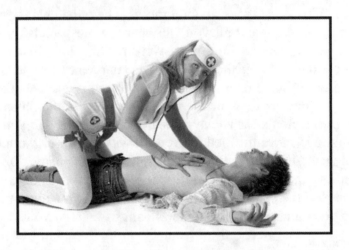

Figure 3: Feel Free to Fantasize

What if you are engaging in the fantasy of being under the boss's desk, giving him a blowjob while you are in real life giving one to your blue collar boyfriend? Is this cheating? Is this wrong? No. Can it feel wrong? Sometimes.

Fantasies Enable Self-Awareness

Some of us may come to realize that our fantasies, the ones that make us red hot, are way beyond anything we might consider acceptable in real life. This could make us feel very uncomfortable, even though we are the only ones who know what we fantasize about. We may attach moral judgments on specific acts that are unfair or unnecessary. Perhaps our "evil" fantasy materializes unbidden while we were making love to our partner. We feel guilty, thinking we wouldn't be having these bad thoughts if we truly loved our partner. It is as if we have cheated on him even though he is clueless.

Be honest here. Just because you love someone doesn't mean that you are immune to everyone else. That would be

Fellatio

unrealistic and ridiculous. It would require that women wear burkas and men wear suits of armor. No one (at least, not in America) wants to do that (unless that happens to be one of your fantasies, in which case, go for it).

How can we make ourselves stop feeling guilty about erotic fantasies? First, we must recognize their advantages. Accept that neither you nor your loved one can actually be hurt by a fantasy. Just because you are fantasizing about having sex or giving fellatio to someone else, does not mean you want to do it in real life. Use fantasy as a tool to make the one you love happier and more fulfilled. Take this opportunity to participate in the activities you are unwilling or unable to perform in actuality. Use it as a learning tool. Gain insights into what makes you the sensual person you truly are. Get to know what turns you on and what turns you off. Try things in your dreams that you would never allow yourself to think about, much less do. Perhaps it might translate into reality in the future, if you are able to expand your horizons.

Fantasy is one of our most powerful sex tools, and it doesn't cost a thing. Use it to heighten pleasure and to aid orgasm. Remember, just because you fantasize about something you consider terrible—for example, being raped by a satyr—doesn't mean you actually want to be raped by a satyr. (If you don't know what a satyr is, check the *Glossary*.) It doesn't mean that you are a bad person (fantasizing, not being ignorant about satyrs). Fantasy is neither good nor bad, so avoid placing moral judgments upon a thought. We all do it. It may not necessarily be of a sexual nature, but we think about what we would do if we won the lottery, or how it would feel to smash in our 13-year-old daughter's boyfriend's smug face.

Pleasure Interrupting Thoughts

While fantasies are generally considered pleasant thoughts, avoid thinking of things during lovemaking that take you away from the moment. Don't spend time worrying about the housework that needs to be done or what to cook for dinner tomorrow night. Tune out the negative, tune in the pleasurable. Caesar Milan, "The Dog Whisperer," says that dogs live in the moment. We need to take a chapter from our dog's book of life, and do the same. When we are giving our significant other a great blowjob, or engaging in any other sexual pleasure, we must stay in the moment. **Don't rob yourself of the joy by being somewhere else when all the fun is happening right where you are now.**

4
How it works: The Anatomy of Male Sexual Arousal

What delights lurk beneath the male of the species' jeans? Most women (or men) reading this probably already know the basics. You know about what you can readily see. But do you know how it works and why? Let's explore male sexuality, beginning with the most obvious.

First, there is a penis. It may or may not be circumcised, but in the United States, chances are that it is. Beneath (or behind) that is the scrotal sack, which contains two testicles. The perineum leads from the balls to the anus. There will be some pubic hair, which covers much of the aforementioned areas. How much depends on your guy and how hairy he is all over.

Those are the things we can see. It all seems pretty simple, doesn't it? But what goes on beneath that skin and muscle and hair? To most of us, it is a complete mystery, despite sex education classes. It is considerably more complex than it appears. Before we begin to explore the inner workings of male genitalia, however, let's examine more closely their outer manifestations.

The Outer Body

Penis

Size. What is a large penis? What constitutes a small penis? In order to answer these questions, we must first know what the average penis measures. In addition, we must make the distinction between whether it is soft or hard. Sticking strictly within the United States of America, penises measure between 2 and 4 inches soft and between 5 and 7 inches erect. The average erect circumference (distance around) is between 4 and 5 inches.

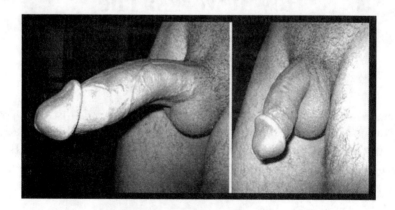

Figure 4: Circumcised Penis, Erect and Unerect

There are other ways to measure penises. In 1993, for example, a study was conducted by the University of Toronto. These particular researchers measured limp penises. They lined up the limp members along rulers placed at the penis's base, then stretched them. This stretching enabled them to obtain a size range for unerect penises. The range was from 2-3/8 inches

Fellatio

to 5-1/4 inches. The average limp penis was 3-3/4 inches. As you can see, stretching the little weenies along a ruler render a bit larger measurement than not stretching them. All this proves regarding the size of penises is that measuring them is not an exact science.

Judging Penises. The great Masters and Johnson discovered that smaller limp penises grew more than their larger counterparts. That is, you cannot use an unerect penis's size to calculate what size it will be when it is erect. Apparently, once they are erect, the smaller ones may catch up with the larger ones, all enlarging to a relatively universal size. Isn't that good news, guys? Ladies?

Never judge the penises you deal with on a day-to-day basis by the ones you see in adult magazines. Just as if they were high-priced fashion models, the photographed penises had all sorts of techniques performed on them—not sexual techniques, but photographic ones. They were airbrushed, washed with flattering light, positioned to show their best side, and angled so that they looked bigger. In addition, some of them are shaved and smeared with makeup, kind of like what we women do before we go to the local photographer.

Shape. Penises come in as many sizes and shapes as there are sizes and shapes of men. Many of them are as straight as your hair after you flatiron it. Some of them are curved. They may go up, down, left, right or any direction in between. When erect, some penises may be firmer at one end than they are at the other. Expect anything when it comes to your fellow's favorite appendage.

Head. The head of the penis contains more nerve endings than any other part of the organ. Obviously, this makes it highly responsive to touch or any type of stimulation. Different guys respond to different stimuli and to varying degrees. The only way to know for sure is to ask your guy if something feels good or if he doesn't like it. Once he has orgasmed, he may be even more sensitive. Pay special attention to his reactions if you want to squeeze him after he has come. Be especially careful with a man who is circumcised. The nerve endings in his penis are more exposed, subjected to constant rubbing from clothes, and therefore highly sensitive.

Uncircumcised. If your man is not circumcised (uncut), the head of his penis will be covered with foreskin. This foreskin, or hood, is made up of skin similar to that covering the rest of the penis. One source compared the inside of this covering to the skin of the inner labia of women. The foreskin, like the hood on your favorite hoodie, moves up and down when it is stimulated by the hand, mouth or vagina.

Frenulum. When a man is circumcised, or had the foreskin cut away from the penis, a V-shaped ridge of skin is left behind. This ridge is called the "frenulum." It is an area that is quite sensitive for many men.

Now, we are ready to follow the shaft of the penis to its base. There you will come upon the scrotum.

Scrotum and Testicles

The scrotum is a soft, wrinkly sack, kind of like linen, which holds the balls, or testicles. Men typically have two testicles unless they have a birth defect, injury or accident. If one testicle is removed or lost, for example, from cancer, most men can function just fine with one. It's the same as with women who function with one ovary.

Perineum

Let's explore further. Once we leave the testicles and scrotum, we arrive at a flat area that is sometimes covered with hair. This skin is often the same color as the penis and is called the "perineum." This area is the so-called root of the penis, which you would know if you had x-ray vision and could see beneath the surface. When a man becomes aroused and gets an erection, the perineum hardens just like his penis does. It has been suggested that, if you rub or stroke this area just as you would his penis, you will be rewarded with a similar response.

The slang or colloquial expression for the perineum is "taint" (see *Glossary*).

Anus

Known by many other names, the anus is the opening at the far end of the perineum from which the man has bowel movements. It is also famous for being sat on all day.

Skin

The other notable organ comprising the man's genitalia is his skin. The skin covering a man's pubic mound, perineum and anus feel quite similar to the skin covering the other parts of his body, but it is normally a different shade. The color may deepen and change at the penis base and scrotum. It becomes darker, softer and thinner than in other areas. This is one of the many reasons these areas are more sensitive to stimulation than other body parts.

Healthy Erections

How does a man achieve and maintain a healthy, consistent erection? Physicians recommend what could be considered obvious: (1) consume a low-fat diet, (2) exercise on a regular basis, (3) keep your weight within standard requirements for health, (4) don't smoke or chew tobacco, and (5) maintain a positive mental attitude.

What Goes on Inside?

The Phases of Erection

The phases of a man's erection can be divided into four parts: arousal, plateau, orgasm and resolution. We will discuss each of these individually below.

Arousal. In order to begin the erection process, the man must become excited about something or someone. Hopefully, what he is excited about is you. If we follow the usual course, sex begins with foreplay. However, there are other methods of getting a man aroused. Reading and watching pornography are among them, but these methods will be discussed later, as will foreplay.

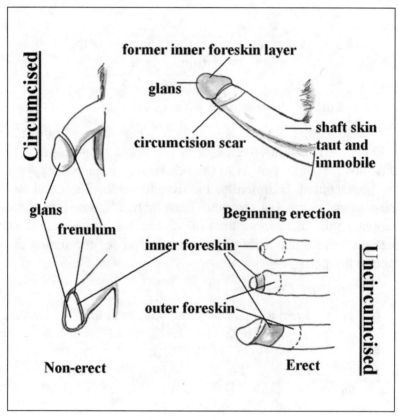

Figure 5: Penis Circumcised and Uncircumcised

An aroused man may leak fluid from the opening of his urethra (see **Glossary**). This fluid serves the purpose of preparing him to come, and is commonly called "pre-come." Pre-come may gush out like water from an opened floodgate, or it may trickle out like a leaky faucet. It is an individual thing, just as a woman's lubricating fluid is. Pre-come will also help lubricate the penis and the vagina, preparing it for intercourse. It is important to remember that pre-come, whether it is mighty or minute, contains the same ingredients as ejaculate. Therefore, it

Fellatio

should be treated exactly the same way. Take all the safe sex precautions that you would take for come. Remember that it is not only possible to get AIDS from pre-come, but you could also become pregnant (if you are a woman, of course).

Plateau. As petting progresses, the man will eventually receive enough stimulation to reach the stage that is called a "plateau." This means that he has reached the high point of his arousal, and that something must happen, and it must happen quickly. As his testicles draw up into his body, the phase comes to an end fairly quickly. After a few minutes, the man passes to the orgasm phase.

Orgasm. In order for the man to orgasm, seminal fluid must pool at the base of the penis. Once it does, and this happens quickly, an orgasm is inevitable. Nothing on earth will prevent it from happening. The muscles propel the semen as it rushes through the penis, bursting forth in the final leg of its journey. Ejaculate squirts out of the penis every 4/5ths of a second. Only after a number of squirts, normally somewhere around four, does the blast begin to taper off.

A man can have an erection without having an ejaculation and vice versa. They can be accomplished independently because each event functions using different nerve pathways.

When blood flows into the tissues and swells them against the skin covering the penis, an erection occurs. If your man is uncircumcised, the swelling pushes the glans (see *Glossary*) out of the opening of the foreskin. If he is circumcised, this step is omitted.

Erections are rarely the same in any two men, and often not the same in one man. They can reach various stages of stiffness: soft, semi-soft, hard or rock hard. As discussed earlier, the size of the penis may change proportionally to its original size. In other words, if it is large when limp, it may not grow much larger when hard. If it is small when limp, it may grow much larger. The size tends to even out when erect. Knowing this fact, we can deduce that large penises may look good, but they are functionally unnecessary.

The man's arousal cycle can peak or valley, and his penis may follow suit. It can grow softer or harder, depending on the length of a particular sexual encounter. This up-and-down cycle has nothing to do with his sexual desire, and is not a reflection on his attraction to his partner. It is merely a part of the process. Neither party to the experience should be concerned about this natural phenomenon.

Everything in his body begins to build to a point where there is no going back. The head of his penis becomes very sensitive, and the entire penis hardens, as does the prostate. As the testicles scrunch close to the body, they create a luscious pressure.

Drugs, which give him an incredible high, are released into his body. Just before he peaks, the prostate gland shudders. It releases its fluid, which mixes with his semen and other juices. At this point there is an "orgasmic inevitability," which cannot be stopped by any power on earth.

When fluids containing ejaculate are forced into the prostatic urethra, the inevitability of orgasm is created. Involuntary orgasmic muscular contractions occur, which alert him that he is about to come. The opening to the bladder is closed and the orgasm begins. Vibrations, contractions and sensations are felt throughout the genital area, not just the penis.

Men expel ejaculate in varying amounts, with an average of 1 to 2 teaspoons. This amount is related to how often he masturbates, participates in fellatio or has intercourse. Stress and other subjective factors may contribute to the variations. Ejaculate is composed of plasma, fluid from the prostate and seminal vesicles, and contains approximately 90 million sperm. The other fluids in ejaculate contain fructose, protein, citric acid, alkaline, and other nutrients that keep sperm intact. The color is whitish, and the texture has been compared to egg whites or hair conditioner. These are all things to keep in mind

Fellatio

if you plan on swallowing it or smearing it in your hair. Sounds like it might be good for either purpose.

As we stated before, semen can be launched out of the penis with the power of a missile or barely trickle out, depending on the guy.

Often, a young or inexperienced guy can suffer from premature ejaculation (see *Glossary*). Control of this process will come with time and experience. It is suggested that using one or even two condoms will decrease the penis's sensitivity and increase the chance of a man being able to hold back. Another method would be more frequent masturbation. Being able to hold back for long periods of time may not be desirable to the party who is giving the fellatio, however.

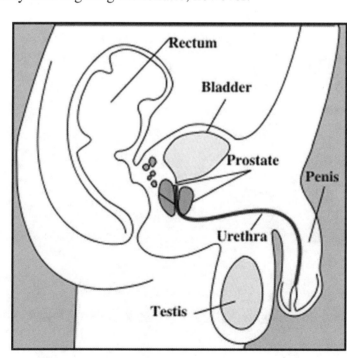

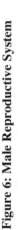

Figure 6: Male Reproductive System

Resolution. After the ejaculation is complete, there is a period of complete relaxation for both the man's body and mind. Its length depends on the man. Common belief is that most of them just roll over and go to sleep immediately. Or is that one of those myths of male sexuality that we have warned you not to believe? Perhaps it is time to lay back and smoke a cigarette. Not really. Smoking can lead to hardening of the arteries, which can lead to the inability to get an erection. We don't want that, do we?

5 Special Spots and Special Issues

Sweet Spot

There is a highly sensitive part of a man's penis that he loves having stimulated in any way. It lies beneath the head of his cock. It may begin at the urethral opening (depending on the man) or farther down, close to the circumcision scar. If the man is uncircumcised, the spot is approximately where the inner skin of the foreskin's hood meets the outer skin of the penis. When making love to a man, specifically when giving him fellatio, pay particular attention to this area. He will be highly grateful.

Prostate

Some people consider the prostate to be the male "G-spot." The man's prostate is an important player in the arousal-to-orgasm phases discussed in the previous chapter. When a man reaches the point of no return, the prostate begins to spasm and contract. It joins the seminal vesicles and other ducts in the process necessary to stimulate orgasm. The man's prostate hardens, just as his penis does. On the outside, it can be felt in the sensitive area between the scrotum and the anus, called the perineum (see *Glossary*).

It is also possible to stimulate the man's prostate from the inside (done through the anus), which he may or may not like. In this situation, you can feel it harden and contract before orgasm.

Anus

Anal stimulation is one of those procedures that some men can't get enough of and some men won't even consider. It's up to you to find out what your man prefers. If he likes his anus penetrated, the process will give you access to the prostate from the inside. This could make the fellatio experience one he is not likely to forget for a long time.

What Special Issues Arise (No Pun Intended)?

We usually think of sex as incorporating the sense of feeling, so it is probably not necessary to discuss its relevance here. However, no communication between a man and a woman stimulates the five senses more than the sex act. It incorporates each of them in a way no other activity can.

Sight

Most Men Are Visual

It is a commonly held belief that most men are visual. This does not mean that they do not use their other senses. It merely means that the primary sense they utilize first and most often is sight. Whether any of the other senses is engaged or not, a man can become aroused immediately upon seeing something that titillates him. It does not necessarily have to be overtly sexual. Just a suggestion of what is available.

This is why it is important that you set the mood for your man before beginning a fellatio session. Pretend you are setting a seductive scene for a movie or play (see **Chapter 1**).

Fellatio

Once the stage is set, and your guy is in a relaxed and receptive position, begin to do a little striptease for him. Take your time and let his eyes take in everything. They will be bugging out of his sockets, and his penis will be doing its best to escape its imprisonment inside his pants.

While you are dancing, here are a few movements and gestures that will make him crazy: squeeze your breasts, tweak your nipples, suck your middle finger and rub it across your pouty lips. Throw your hair over your head, and back and forth across your face. Get into the feeling of the dance, and give it all your enthusiasm.

I can already hear what you are thinking: I am too fat; he will think I look stupid. Rest assured, those thoughts will not be going through your guy's head during your dance, so you should banish them from your mind also.

The Star of Fellatio

Your mouth will be the star during fellatio, and he won't be able to keep his eyes off of what you are doing to him. It would be nice if your lips remained ripe and red through the whole process. Many men would love that. However, as we all know, keeping lipstick on is a difficult business, regardless of whether it is coming off during the administration of fellatio. It comes off on teeth, on straws and everything else it comes in contact with. A theatrical makeup called "Lip Set" by Signature Solutions or Cover Girl's Outlast lipstick may solve the problem. However, Cover Girl still tests their products on animals, and we shouldn't give pleasure at the expense of someone else's pain.

34   The Sensuous Couple's Guide to Seismic Oral Sex

When you've really got your guy going, surprise him by quickly raising your head and looking him directly in the eye. It will blow his mind. If you aren't brave enough for the eyeball-to-eyeball approach, try glancing at him coyly from the corner of your eye. If you do it at significant times during the blowjob, he will be sure to notice.

Sound

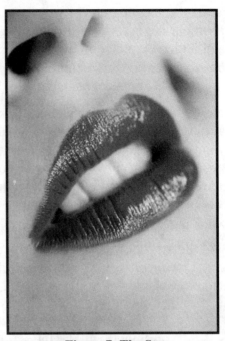

Figure 7: The Star

Men are stimulated by sound, second only to vision. Some of them may have a special song they like to listen to while making love. They might have a different one for fellatio sessions. Check with your partner to see if he has a selection. Remember Bo Derek in *10*? She made Dudley Moore restart Ravel's *Bolero* several times before their love-making session (which never actually materialized). You will have your mouth full, so don't try to sing along. Humming would be good, though. Really make his penis vibrate!

Murmurs, groans, moans, mumbling, humming—almost any sound you make during fellatio will turn your man on even more. Don't forget our advice in Chapter 1. Repeat his name as often as you can think to do it. The sound of his own name is better music to his ears than his favorite fellatio tune.

Smell

As you would expect, cleanliness is very important when engaging in fellatio. Always bathe, and make sure your

Fellatio

partner has bathed also. Pay close attention to the genital area. The man should take special precautions when he is anticipating a blowjob, particularly if he is not circumcised. He wants to be pristine when he is anticipating his partner going down on him.

Generally, a man's genital area is going to both taste and smell the same way he tastes and smells elsewhere. If you already love the way he smells, you are not going to have much trouble engaging in a tête-à-tête with his penis. It may be a bit more musky, salty or tangy due to pre-come. This is a good thing, because pre-come arrives in a package crammed with chemicals and pheromones that are calculated to turn on the other party. There is a possibility he may not smell the same way every time, but it will be close enough.

A man's smell may be influenced by many factors, which are discussed in the "Taste" section below.

Taste

Taste is the same as smell. It depends on many factors. You may not be quite as concerned about it, however, unless you plan to allow your partner to ejaculate into your mouth.

While it is true that pre-come contains most of the elements that ejaculate does, it is not released in the same quantity nor with the same force. Both of these issues may be factors in determining whether or not to allow him to ejaculate in your mouth.

Taste of Ejaculate

All men's come varies somewhat in taste. Most likely, if you have already decided you love his allover taste (and smell), you will feel the same way about his ejaculate. What attracts some people to one person and not another must be chemical, since there is no other way of accounting for it. Whatever mysterious chemistry one man has that turns you on may not be palatable for another woman, and vice versa. Do you hold his pillow to your nose or wear his shirt around the house after he's gone? If you do, then chances are you will be amenable to handling the taste of his ejaculate.

Pre-come is a preview of how his come will taste. If you need a larger sample, it has been suggested that you allow him to come in your hand, or on another body part, then taste a bit of the come on your fingertips. Do not let your man see you do this. If you decide, based on this sample, that you do not want him to come in your mouth, then his feelings may be hurt. Men are sensitive about their come, as they want the taste to be pleasant to you. If it is not, they may feel humiliated. It is always better to be thoughtful.

What Affects the Taste of Come?

Pungent Semen. Here are a few flavors that allegedly make semen taste strong or pungent: vitamins, asparagus, beets, onions, broccoli, cauliflower, coffee, cigarettes, alcohol and garlic. These things can affect the semen the same way they can affect a man's urine. If he wants to keep his ejaculate neutral, he should avoid the listed substances for 24 hours before engaging in oral sex. He should also drink plenty of fresh water, which serves to neutralize the urine and semen.

Carnivore vs. Vegetarian. Strictly speaking, humans are NEVER carnivorous. A carnivore only eats meat. If meat were the only so-called food humans devoured, they would die very soon. Men who eat greater quantities of meat than they do plant-based materials will have stronger tasting semen than vegetarians. Is this unpleasant? Not necessarily. It depends on the person who is doing the tasting.

Who can forget the episode of the *Sex in the City* when Samantha's latest sexy professional, Adam, was great except for the "funky tasting spunk" (possibly because he ate too much meat), and Samantha refused to perform oral sex on him?

For the record, none of the sources I read suggest any animal-based product as a come-sweetener. All suggestions were plant-based. Apparently, having a fruit salad before sex might be the best turn-on a man could do. The come-sweeteners suggested were: strawberries, sweet melons, papaya, mango, raspberries, blueberries, pineapple, any citrus or celery juice. Whether this really works or not, it would be fun to try and would be good for his health also. Maybe he could eat the fruit salad off your breasts or tummy.

Products. There are commercial substances that claim to change the taste of semen, but we do not recommend them. They have passed no clinical or safety trials, and they assume that semen tastes bad in the first place. The majority of us probably don't really think that anyway. We probably want to taste our partner the way he really tastes, not the way some corporation thinks he should taste.

To Swallow or Not to Swallow

That IS the Question

Whether to direct the ejaculate to a predetermined spot that is as far away from your mouth as possible, or to let it land squarely in your mouth and swallow it with the same gusto you would a piece of chocolate cake—that is the question.

As with all things sexual, it depends on the individuals involved. There are some people who feel neutral, others who can't wait to swallow their beloved's semen, and those who find the idea quite distasteful.

Pre-Established Signal. If you are the male receiving the blowjob, please consult your partner before you let go inside the private sanctity of their mouth. The two of you should have established a specific procedure to take before the actual event is upon you. If the person giving the fellatio does not want the man to come in their mouth, then come up with a pre-established signal. When the signal is enacted, it is a warning that the man is about to ejaculate. The signal could be anything: a tap on the shoulder, a playful yank of the hair, the man could withdraw himself before he begins to orgasm, or anything that you two agree upon.

Why Wouldn't Someone Want to Swallow? Oral sex is considered to be the most intimate of all sexual encounters. Most likely, this is not something we are going to be doing with someone we hardly know (especially if we are the giver). Regardless of how permissive our society appears to have become, we are still descended from Puritans. If you compare American sexual attitudes to those of Europeans, we always appear much less sophisticated about it than they do. Sex is shameful for many; the genitals are dirty; oral sex is a degrading taboo. At the present time, our country seems to be as polarized on this subject as we are on political matters. One group wants less sex; the other group wants more. Perhaps your attitude is somewhere in the middle.

Emotional Needs of Men

The cult of the supermodel makes every average woman reluctant to show her body. The images of perfection keep us from sharing ourselves in intimate ways for fear of not being beautiful or good enough. This is true for men as well as women. Men may think their bodies aren't sexy enough, or they may not smell or taste good. He may be afraid of not giving a perfect performance.

If you care about your partner, you may want to give him a blowjob to show your affection, to share the most intimate of acts with him. Due to the length of your relationship, you may have already developed the prerequisite trust necessary. If your relationship is of short duration, it will take some time to build up the necessary trust.

Some experts suggest that you keep a washcloth handy in case the man does not want to be kissed after you have had his genitals in your mouth. Is it okay for you to have it in YOUR mouth, but not okay for him? Conversely, is it acceptable for him to kiss you after he has gone down on you? All of us are individuals with individual desires and limitations. You and your partner might want to reassess your ideas of what is dirty and what isn't.

6 Getting Started

Psychology

Difference between Mental and Physical

The physical act of oral sex is pretty straightforward. The psychological aspects may be somewhat more complicated. We will discuss them both so that the reader will become comfortable with each aspect.

Physical. Having another person touch your genitals with something other than their hand is the physical act of oral sex. Fellatio, specifically, means having someone else touch a man's penis with their mouth in such a way as to cause a reaction. This reaction is the blood flowing into the penis which causes the penis to harden.

Mental. What is the mental aspect of oral sex? There is a pathway that leads directly from a man's brain to his penis. Sights, sounds or fantasies can trigger this mechanism, just the same as being touched. The same result is accomplished. The blood flows into his penis, and he has an erection.

The First Time

It is only natural to have insecurities when it is your first time. This holds true whether you are the one giving the blowjob or the one receiving it. Either of you may be asking yourself: Will I do it right? Will I be good enough? How long will it take? What do I do if he doesn't come? On and on this goes until you can drive yourself crazy.

This is one of those times when it is best not to think too much. You have read this book and others, so just allow the knowledge you have absorbed to float to the surface as it is needed.

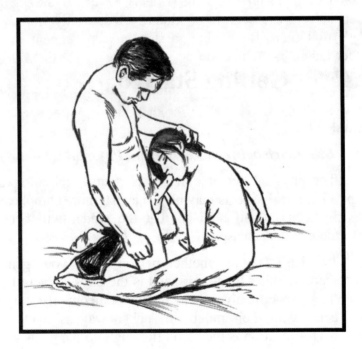

Figure 8: The First Time

If you are the man receiving the blowjob, the fear of not being able to get an erection may be the cause of your stress. If you tell yourself this often enough, you may convince your brain that it is true. It will become a self-fulfilling prophecy.

Fellatio

The neural highway that transverses the brain and the penis may be difficult to access if we are obscuring the path with negative thinking. Take the same advice we are giving the kind person who is giving you the blowjob. DO NOT THINK. Too much thinking is a wreck caused by you that blocks the road. There are no alternate routes. As the receiver, all you really need to do is lie back and relax. Let your partner do the rest. Whatever they decide to do, most likely, will be enjoyable. The partner will communicate with you (either before or during the fellatio). That is the time to express your needs and wants.

There is one overt act that the receiver can do, however. Be encouraging, supporting and patient with the giver. Dig deep to tap into your reservoir of kindness, especially if it is the giver's first time. Be willing to stop at any moment if your partner indicates the need to do so. Do not berate them if they are unable to finish. You can finish yourself, or they can aid you with a hand job. The next time, things will go more smoothly. They will be more than willing to try again if you treated them with kindness and patience.

Why Men Have Difficulty Getting and Maintaining Erections

Every man, at one time or another, will have some difficulty achieving and/or maintaining an erection. Perfectly understandable. Not understandable are the 30,000,000 men, as reported by the National Institutes of Health, who consistently have trouble in this area. A large, sad figure.

There are numerous reasons for this problem. The most common reason is the use of drugs, both legal and illegal. Physicians prescribe drugs for a number of ailments (all ailments, actually, since that is what an allopathic doctor is trained to do). They are doled out for mental problems, such as stress, anxiety, depression and substance abuse (seems like an oxymoron). Other health conditions for which doctors give drugs and can cause impotence are arteriosclerosis, diabetes, high cholesterol and high blood pressure. The list goes on ad infinitum: low testosterone from age or HIV; neurological issues caused by accidents, surgery, MS or Parkinson's, prostate conditions or smoking. Here's a suggestion: take care of yourself and you won't need prescription drugs, and you won't malfunction.

The Power Dynamic of Fellatio

Who is in Control? It depends on who you are asking. Many people feel that a certain dynamic is inherent to fellatio— whoever is receiving the blowjob is the powerful one. They allege that the person giving the blowjob is the submissive one. This attitude could arise from the fact that it is usually a woman who is the giver. They are considered by some to be the weaker sex. While this attitude has received quite a beating since the days of women's liberation, it is persistently with us even to this day. Also, the person who is the giver is in what some might consider a submissive position. They may perceive the receiver as actually "giving" or "putting" it to her, thus giving him the dominant role. When examined more closely, this dynamic doesn't ring true. It is really the person who is performing the fellatio who is "giving" it to him. By that definition, they would be in control.

Changing Control. If you are the giver, and you consider yourself in the submissive role, perhaps you would like to change the dynamic. This will require cooperation from the receiver. He must agree to refrain from doing anything that might intimidate the giver. One such move would be grabbing the back of the giver's head and forcing it forward onto his penis. Another one would be violently jabbing his penis into the mouth of the giver. Such moves could cause the giver to become scared. They may gag, and want to stop giving the fellatio. If you are the receiver, do not force them to continue, even if you are near orgasm. It may be uncomfortable for you, but it is better to allow the giver leeway in performing the task as best suits them.

Fellatio

They may have to switch to a hand job because of muscle fatigue. However, such a switch in the action could possibly lead to a more forceful orgasm. The giver will be very grateful for the rest, and this will make them more willing to do it again—a happy event for all involved.

The change in position—from blowjob to hand job—can help change the dynamic. If the giver wants to, they can try blindfolding the receiver, use pain, sex toys or playacting to maintain control over the activity. Ideally, the couple will have discussed these things beforehand.

Can We Unlearn Negative Attitudes About Sex?

In many cultures, the person who is willing to allow a man to put his penis in their mouth is considered dirty and undeserving. They believe that fellatio is exclusively for the benefit of the receiver. The giver is merely the vessel used to accomplish the deed. The giver, it is perceived, derives no pleasure from the deed, just as a machine does not enjoy its job.

For many people, this is patently untrue. Becoming aroused, getting wet and actually having an orgasm while performing fellatio is not uncommon. Some women claim to reach orgasm from going down on a man, requiring no physical stimulation either from her partner or herself.

The idea that the sex organs are dirty, and not to be seen or touched, usually stems from childhood teachings and attitudes forced upon us by our parents and elders. It is often difficult to overcome these feelings when we become adults. To deal with this pesky problem—aside from receiving years of psychoanalysis— begin by being as clean as possible before we perform the act.

Cleanliness

Daily Showering

It is absolutely necessary to shower every day, a practice that seems to be commonplace among Americans. Perhaps other countries will follow suit, just as they are duplicating other American customs. If you are an uncircumcised man, be sure to pull back the foreskin of the penis, and scrub thoroughly. Before fellatio, the two of you could take a shower (or bubble bath) together. Soap each other down, and you will already be "up" for the event that is to come.

It has been suggested that "rimmers" (see **Glossary**) be especially careful about cleanliness. Some men may even want to take an enema beforehand. Most of us had rather not, however. Try eating plenty of fiber in the form of fruits, vegetables and whole grains, and you will always be clean on the inside.

Pubic Hair

Dealing with It. Feeling a tickle at the back of your throat? Pubic hair does exist, and we cannot avoid it. The question is, how do we get around it?

Some guys are cavemen when it comes to hair, some are babies. Then, there are those that vary between these two extremes. It seems as if the less hair they have on the top of their heads, the more hair they have covering every other part of their bodies. As a general rule, pubic hair begins at a man's navel. It leaves a trail of fuzz that can extend to his pubic bone. It then surrounds the base of his penis while stretching over his testicles and scrotum. It can even spread as far down as the top of a man's thighs. Their butt crack may often be furry.

This may sound unsavory, I admit, but when you are in the throes of sexual passion, most likely the amount of hair will cease to matter. If not, keep thinking about your favorite sexual fantasy actor. It will make things easier.

Shaving. The benefits of shaving are a mixed bag. Most men have never bothered to shave the genital area of their bodies. They may not realize that their skin becomes all the more sensitive because of this, and for that reason alone it may be worth it.

Fellatio

Keep in mind, however, that when the hair starts to grow back, which is very soon, the area begins to itch. It quickly becomes stubble, just like on your face. One possibility is that when the stubble appears, shave again or cover the area with a small towel to prevent your lover from receiving beard burn. However, that is adding another item to an already complicated mix of soaping and showering within an inch of your life, using a condom (hopefully), and God knows what other protections and devices. Do you really need to add "a small towel" to the mix?

More importantly, do you really want to add another area to your daily shaving ritual? Take it from women, shaving is a pain, especially when you have several areas to cover. It used to be just the underarms and legs. Now it is the pubic area. It seems like every woman wants to look like a little girl again and get rid of every ounce of hair on their bodies.

Shaving Suggestions. That's fine, but most women prefer their men to look like adults, not like hairless boys. If you still insist on trying the shaving routine, here are a few hints about how to do it more effectively:

1. Treat the area you are about to shave the way you would a full beard. First, use small scissors to trim the hair. Make sure your scissors and razor are sharp.
2. Put some bath oil in your bath water, or rub it into your skin before you shower. Shave while you are in the shower or the bathtub. Both of these methods will soften the hair.
3. Lather up with a moisturizing shaving cream or gel. Products that are specifically made for shaving will work better than bar soap.
4. If you use disposable razors, change them often.
5. Shave the same direction as the hair grows, just as you would with your beard.

6. The testicles and scrotum are very delicate areas. To ensure their safety, use your fingers to stretch the wrinkly skin out flat before you use a blade on it. (Just typing that made me nervous.)
7. Apply a hypoallergenic lotion to the shaved area, which will help prevent itching when it begins to grow out. Avoid powder; it dries the skin.
8. Use a cortisone cream to treat razor burn or excessive itching. Do not use it more than twice weekly. It can cause the skin to thin.

Woman Shaving a Man. If you want to shave your man yourself, the first step is to have him sit on a towel while maintaining a stable position. Be sure you have access to running water or have a bowl of warm water available. Shave all the parts you have immediate access to. Leave the delicate parts—like his balls—to him. You wouldn't want to be responsible for cutting or severing one of his vital organs.

Just remember that, regardless of who is doing the shaving, it will grow back, start to itch and must be shaved again.

Waxing. If you thought shaving was a mini-horror show, wait until you hear about waxing. Why do men put themselves through this ordeal? Perhaps they are models, porn stars, swimmers or bodybuilders who compete. I suggest you have a really good reason for doing the following:

Warm wax is placed on the area where hair is to be removed and allowed to cool. It is then ripped away. If you have seen *The 40-Year-Old Virgin*, you can tell it hurts like hell! But that's not all. Waxing most likely did not get all the little culprits, so it's once-over with the tweezers. Have you ever tried to pull out pubic hair with tweezers? Holy Excruciating Agony, Batman! Then the waxing attendant gets the wrong idea, because low and behold, you have an erection. Not because you are turned on, but because the pain stimulates blood flow and nerve endings. Your erection is your body's response to the stimulation. The attendant thinks you actually enjoyed the whole experience. The embarrassing truth is that you just want to curl up in a fetal position, suck your thumb and cry for mommy.

You stay red, swollen and quite sore for a few days. You stay hairless (more or less) for up to six weeks. "I'm free!" you think, but how long is six weeks in the overall scheme of things? There's a good possibility that you will be constantly thinking about and dreading that next waxing the entire six weeks!

Perhaps, you think, you could wax at home, and it would be less painful and cheaper. Don't do it! It is better to let a professional do this. How good of a job are you going to do anyway, when it means causing yourself pain? The professional is trained to hurt you and won't let you off the hook until you are skinned like the serial killer victims in *The Silence of the Lambs*.

Laser Removal. Hair removal lasers have been in use since 1997 for permanent hair reduction. Both men and women use laser hair removal services to have unwanted hair removed. It has become extremely popular because of its speed and efficacy, although both are dependent on the skill and experience of the laser operator, and the availability of different laser technology at the clinic which is performing the procedure.

Hair removal is commonly done on upper lips, chin, ear lobe, shoulders, back, underarm, abdomen, buttocks, pubic area, bikini lines, thighs, face, neck, chest, arms, legs, hands, and toes. Laser works best with dark coarse hair. Light skin and dark hair are an ideal combination, but new lasers are now able to target dark black hair even in patients with dark skin. Some will need touch-up treatments, especially on large areas, after the initial set of 3-8 treatments.

Communication

We have our positive mental attitude in place, we are scrubbed down and pristine, so now we are ready to commence fellatio. Right?

Not quite yet. This may be a stressful time, and the best way to alleviate some of that tension is to listen to how the other person is feeling. Chances are, they are as nervous and apprehensive as you are.

Open up a line of communication with your partner. Give them ample opportunity to tell you what is on their minds—positive and negative. Talking about sex enhances the act; it doesn't diminish it. If your partner, whether the giver or the receiver, is reluctant, read an erotic story aloud that contains a fellatio scene. Or read him sections from this book. Or let him read them for himself. If you are anxious to extend your sex life and show your confidence and enthusiasm, the other party will soon come around to your way of thinking. Your reassurance will help them become more comfortable with their body and sexuality.

This cannot be repeated enough: Always use a condom when performing or receiving oral sex. The only exception to this would be a very long-term relationship that you are POSITIVE is monogamous and both parties have been tested for STDs. If you use a condom, the giver won't have to worry about whether to allow him to come in your mouth, or whether to swallow or not. That problem will automatically be solved. If you are not using a condom—and you better have a really good reason why you're not—then communicate beforehand a signal that lets you know he is about to come. This is crucial so that you won't be taken by surprise, make a hideous face and hurt his feelings. A tap on the shoulder will suffice.

Fellatio

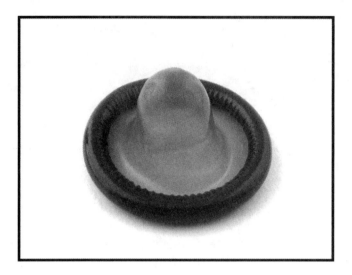

Figure 9: Condom

Experimentation

Practice. Reading books, watching videos and talking about the act of fellatio can make it all much less intimidating. It has also been suggested that you practice on something else before you do the real thing, like a dildo, a cucumber or a zucchini. Don't let him catch you doing this, or he'll wonder why you are assaulting dinner.

Study the anatomy sections of this book so you will know what you are feeling and what his body is experiencing.

Try grazing, nuzzling, kissing and pressing your tongue into the hollow of your hand. This will give you an idea of how fellatio feels to him. Practice using different strokes and pressures. Put two fingers into your mouth and suck; move them in and out. Basically, experiment doing all the things that you would do if it were his penis in your mouth. This will give you a few tried-and-true techniques that are sure to please him.

7 Technique – Make it Seismic!

General

There is a basic technique for fellatio. The person who is giving the head puts the penis of the person who is receiving it into their mouth, normally while holding it vertical with one or both hands. They then proceed to use their mouth and, to a greater or lesser extent, their hands, to bring the receiver to orgasm. He may ejaculate inside the mouth or not, depending on the wishes of the giver.

Begins with an Erection

Does a man need an erection in order for fellatio to commence? Not necessarily. He may not start out with one. The receiver may begin with a flaccid member, which would actually be better if he is particularly large. It is much easier to take a limp penis into your mouth than it is a hard one. The man has no real control over his erection; that, and his orgasm, depend on what you do to him to get him to that point.

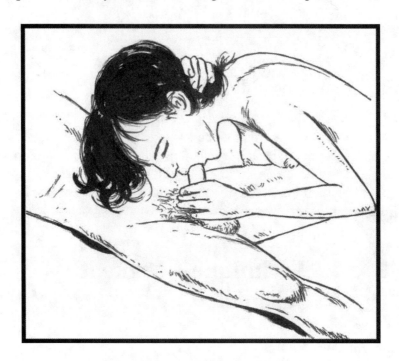

Figure 10: Basic Technique

Doesn't look all that complicated, does it? It's not. But there are a world of variations and techniques that will enhance the experience and make it unique every time, if the partners choose to employ them.

In this chapter, we will address each body part of the giver, and describe its function in the fellatio experience.

Getting Started

If he is dressed, or still has his briefs on, you might begin by mouthing his penis and balls through the fabric. This would give you an introduction to the real thing, and buy you some extra time to get used to the feeling. This also feels great

Fellatio

to the receiver. Once you are ready to move on, help him remove his underwear. You will be face-to-face with his penis. The big moment has arrived, so give yourself a few seconds to adjust, while savoring it at the same time.

What if his penis is pierced? I believe he should have told you about this before you began, but perhaps he thought it would be more exciting if it was a surprise.

As long as the piercing is completely healed, it is really just the same as a pierced ear (well, not exactly), and is perfectly clean. There are many men who pierce their penises and women who enjoy giving fellatio to a man with a pierced penis. The piercing allegedly makes him more sensitive. You will have to observe how he reacts to whatever you do to him, to see if it is feeling okay. Possibly, he merely wants you to ignore it and just allow it to do its job. If it comes out, don't freak. Just let him deal with it.

Hands

Using Hands Before Fellatio. There are numerous things the giver can do with their hands before, during or after placing the penis in their mouth. These techniques will enhance the fellatio experience for the receiver as well as the giver.

By inserting your finger into the man's mouth and allowing him to suck it, you will be giving him a preview of imminent events. The exception is that it will be the reverse of what he will be experiencing.

Make a point to play with his balls (be careful; they can be delicate).

Rub, pinch and squeeze his nipples.

Caress his butt cheeks. The buttocks are highly sensitive but are often ignored. His crack and anus are great areas to administer to, if both of you are willing.

Wrap your hands around his penis, applying enough pressure to emulate the snugness of the vagina. It will feel warm and familiar to him. When you sense that he is close to climax, glide your hand over the coronal ridge, the V-spot and the head. Don't overdo the head, however, as it tends to be uber-sensitive. If you rub it too hard, it can be painful.

Hand Job Grips. Since most blowjobs begin with the hands, below are a few grips that might make the job go easier. These are in no way comprehensive. There are numerous hand job strokes to help him achieve orgasm, but this book is specifically about fellatio. Therefore, we do not go into detail regarding that subject. You can find plenty of information about hand jobs in other books and materials.

A few hand job grips:

1. "OK"—touch index or middle finger to thumb and slip around shaft.
2. "Thank U"—cradle penis in "U" between thumb and fingers.
3. "Sausage Wrap"—enclose shaft in five fingers with thumb at top and stroke.
4. "Upside-Down Sausage Wrap"—reposition wrist so thumb is at bottom of shaft.

Hands Are Extension of Mouth. Your hands can be used to compliment your mouth during fellatio. Without help, your mouth would give out long before he reached a climax. Use your hands in conjunction with your mouth to encompass more of his member. The two of them together create a tunnel (emulating the vagina). He may slide his penis in and out of it. This technique puts the giver in control of his thrusting. It protects the giver from the man becoming too excited and wanting to shove too far or too fast. Substitute the hand if your jaw becomes tired and give it a short rest.

Fellatio

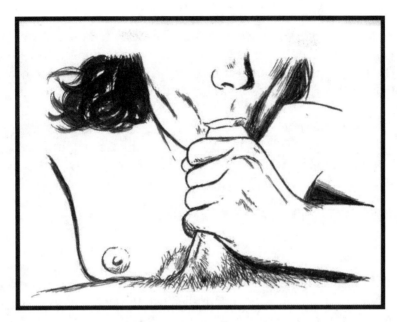

Figure 11: Using the Hand

Mouth

Oral Fixation. People who are smokers or compulsive overeaters tend to be orally fixated. This can be an advantage in fellatio, since the mouth is one of our most potent sex organs. Having his penis in your mouth is visually stimulating to the person who is receiving the blow job. Having his penis in your mouth creates sensations in you that increase your desire. It creates a connection between your pleasure and his.

When I was quitting smoking, my ex-husband used to wag his penis at me and say, "If you need something to suck on, try this." It must have helped. I haven't smoked in many years.

Dental Hygiene. As we have stated previously, much of what turns a man on is visual. Therefore, be sure you have a healthy, clean-looking mouth. Both your teeth and gums need to be sparkling and disease-free. Your breath should smell and taste sweet. You could apply a soft lip balm to make your lips look luscious, or try one of the lipsticks mentioned earlier.

After spending so much time and attention on your teeth, you might think they would be used in fellatio. However, it is best to keep them out of the way when giving a blowjob. I'm not suggesting you get dentures so you can take them out and put them in a glass of water on the bedside table. Although the molars are generally in a safe position, the front teeth can cause some serious damage. The way to cover the front teeth is to seal your mouth over them while keeping lips slightly tensed or pursed. This is rather automatic when you begin giving fellatio, so you won't really have to think about it. Just something to be aware of. There are a few men who might enjoy a light nibbling from your teeth, but this needs to be done with care.

The muscles that control our faces allow us to purse our lips, slacken our jaws and wiggle our tongues. We can lick lollypops or suck a chocolate milkshake through a straw. These are all transferable skills. Use them to enhance your fellatio session; your lover's penis will be most grateful.

Large Penis. Perhaps you are lucky (or unlucky, depending on your point of view), and your guy has a large penis. It may be so large that you are unable to put it all in your mouth at once. This would be the time to use your hands as an extension of your mouth, which would help you contain the entire penis within your control.

Tongue

Our tongue is the most important member of our mouth family. It is the primary organ used to distinguish between all the flavors we are able to taste. The way we taste things is through a combination of effects—smell, touch, texture and temperature. Our tongue can explore the taste of our lover, all the time sending erotic impulses to our brains.

Once you have introduced his penis to your mouth, it is time to begin licking and fluttering your tongue against its head. From the head, move gradually down the shaft.

Fellatio

What is the most neglected area during fellatio? Your vagina, you might say. I mean, what area of the man receiving the fellatio is most often neglected? His testicles or balls. For most men, they are a highly erotic area. If you want to give your man the ultimate pleasure, be sure to pay plenty of attention to them.

Once you have arrived at the base of his penis, linger there to lick his testicles. They are quite sensitive and tender, however, so be careful. Depending on how well you know the man, you should touch them lightly at first, increasing pressure as he responds favorably. Some effective movements are: squeezes and tugs (go easy), fingertip caresses, reaching behind them and stroking the perineum (see *Glossary*). Prolong this kind of approach for as long as you can. Then, very carefully lift his balls and lick the perineum. Pay close attention to his reactions to each of these areas. You will quickly learn which ones are his favorites. Try a trick called "tea bagging." This is the name for the process of sucking his balls into your mouth and holding them there until he cries for mercy.

I am including a few suggestions for using your tongue, if you happen to run out of your own ideas. You have detected where his most sensitive spots are by observation. Flicker your tongue against those places again and again. Another movement is to press your tongue flat against the head of his penis. Also, point your tongue, soften your tongue, and vary licking speeds. Use these guidelines, and it will be rare for you to run out of movements before the session ends.

If his body language is not giving you enough clues as to what he likes the best, and the moans and groans and grunts coming from his mouth aren't helping much either, you might just ask him. (Probably a good idea to take his penis out of your mouth when you do this, as he may not understand the question.) He could answer your question directly.

Basic Stroke

Master Stroke. Place your hand around the base of the penis and your lips over its head. With your hand touching your lips, begin to go up and down on the penis. There are ways you can vary this procedure: use long as opposed to short strokes, go slow or go fast, adjust the pressure of your hand on his penis, or vary the suction of your mouth.

Variations. Use your tongue to create a vacuum. Why do you want to create a vacuum? Because it creates a highly desirable sensation for the penis. Another way to create a vacuum is to constrict your throat and pull with your lips. Hold your mouth still and move your hand up and down, or do just the opposite. A variation on this technique is to twist your head if the hand is still, or twist your hand if the head is still. Other variations would include keeping your tongue constantly moving, or holding still and allowing the man to thrust his penis in your mouth (called "Irrumation"—see *Glossary*).

Gagging

Inevitability. Gagging is an issue that invariably comes up when discussing fellatio. Everyone gags at some point during a blowjob (except the receiver). What causes gagging? It begins when the penis activates nerves in the back of the mouth and the soft palate. Convulsions begin, and the opening to the throat constricts, sending pulses racing to the stomach. Your stomach tightens and pitches, and you become queasy. All of this is a good thing, however. It enables the body to protect itself from choking and/or swallowing oversized objects—like your honey's extra large member, for example.

If we were snakes, we could swallow something bigger than the size of our throats. Unlike them, however, we cannot unhinge our jaws. Our boyfriends might be glad about this, since their penises might be forever lost like that little rabbit going down the rattlesnake's throat. Happily, however, it is possible to overcome gagging.

Fellatio

Overcoming Gagging. Overcoming gagging is possible, but is it desirable? The question is, do we really want to overcome this involuntary reaction? Isn't it for our protection? Isn't it a natural safeguard that we might want to keep intact? Well, yes. But, we never lose it completely. We can overcome it temporarily by staying cool, calm and collected. We can become more comfortable with oral sex and practice certain techniques to overcome it. There will be more about this phenomenon when we discuss "deep throating."

Stroking and Rhythm

In the beginning, when the two of you have not indulged in fellatio very often, limit your strokes to two or three that you know he loves. Instead of switching back and forth quickly among these strokes, establish a slow, methodical rhythm. Stick with one for so many beats, then, predictably, switch to another. Continue that stroke for the same amount of time you did the previous one. Surprise or variety is not necessarily a good thing when he is near orgasm. Keeping it steady and using exactly what you know makes him come is usually the best course. Later, you may add more variety as you are able to read his body's responses, or he may tell you he prefers more variety.

Soon, he should be close to the point of no return. You have, or should have, established a rhythm that is smooth and effective. Don't frustrate him with too many quick tricks. He is concentrating on the ultimate goal, his orgasm, and does not need to be distracted.

On the other hand, he may be getting too wild in his responses. He might be grabbing your hair and pushing your head onto his penis. He might try to grind his pelvis into your face, or grab your ears and force you forward. If this is the case, simply remove his hands and place them onto your shoulders or his own hips. It is better, however, to discuss this beforehand. You may tell him that you prefer to be in charge of the session, and that his attempting to force you to do anything during fellatio makes you uncomfortable. He will respect your wishes.

If he does get a little carried away, it won't be intentional. It will be because you are doing such a sensational job he can't help himself. In this case, he merely needs a gentle reminder.

Getting Tired and Sore

The Giver. Use pillows to position yourself comfortably before you begin the fellatio session. Make sure you do not have to hold your head up the entire time. Place a pillow under his buttocks for easier access. Even with these precautions, most likely your jaw will grow tired after a while. Your neck, or some other body part may begin to ache. When this happens, and it will, change positions. This is perfectly acceptable, and the receiver will understand. Substitute your hand for your mouth, if you have to stop for a few minutes. If it gives you some relief, lick his balls, kiss his thighs or introduce a sex toy. Once you are rested, go back to the rhythmic stroking you had established before.

The Receiver. Even the person who would seem to be the most relaxed — the person receiving the blowjob — can become sore. His foreskin is quite tender, as are his balls. Take it easy when you move the foreskin up and down the penis shaft during stroking. The skin is thin and susceptible to sensory overload. Likewise, the balls can be handled too roughly. To get some idea of the kind of pressure he would like applied to his balls, have him squeeze one of your breasts using the same pressure.

Anus and Internal

Anal Stimulation

Once you have tried all the more common techniques to bring your man to the ultimate orgasm through fellatio, you might want to try something his isn't expecting — anal stimulation. You may have never even considered touching his anus. It is indirectly being stimulated, however, during your lovemaking session, whether you realize it or not. Once a man begins to get worked up, his anus becomes highly sensitive. It

Fellatio 61

will pulsate every time he orgasms, although he may not be totally aware of these sensations himself. If you begin to touch him there, it will heighten his awareness, and he will enjoy it even more.

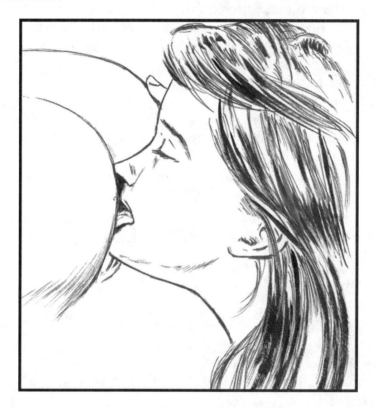

Figure 12: Rimming

Rimming

If you are so inclined, using your tongue around his anus will put him into throes of ecstasy. This activity is the prelude to penetration, so lick and flutter your tongue in and around the area for as long as you can. After performing this act for a short time, penetrate the anus opening with your tongue. This process is called "rimming." Although it can be a source of amazing pleasure, one or both of you may find it distasteful. Take your time, and be sure to discuss it before-hand.

Prostate Stimulation

The prostrate is sometimes referred to as the male "G-spot." The first step to locating and stimulating it is penetration. Using a well-lubricated finger, penetrate the anus and locate the prostate. Once you have found the right spot, crook your finger and stroke forward, as if you were telling some one to "come here." As we have noted previously, the prostrate can be indirectly massaged on the outside. The technique would be to massage the perineum with your thumb. If he didn't like that (and I'm assuming you tried it before you approached penetration), he may not like internal stimulation either. Check for his responses to either technique.

Being able to orgasm by mere anal stimulation is rare. You must continue using your fellatio techniques in order to bring him to orgasm.

Premature Ejaculation

I'm not sure premature ejaculation is a bad thing when you are administering a blowjob. I guess it depends upon whether you are the one giving the blowjob or the one receiving it. In any case, below is a technique to prevent this, if you have a mind to. I guess you've already given him a blowjob, or you wouldn't know he was a premature ejaculator.

With you thumb positioned on the underside, place your hand on the tip of his penis. Your fingertips should be on either side of the coronal ridge and pressing the frenulum (see **Glossary**). When you sense that he is getting close to orgasm (see below for how to know this), squeeze for a few seconds, then quickly release. His erection should subside a little. Wait for approximately 30 seconds, then continue what you were doing. Squeeze him several more times during the fellatio session until you are ready for him to come.

Orgasm and Ejaculation

How Do You Know He Is about to Come?

The man will climax when you have repeated his favorite routines enough times. There are many signs, both physical and verbal. He may moan or yell. I dated a guy who was so loud, I was sure the other people in the motel could hear him. Physically, the muscles in his thighs, jaw, abdomen, hands and feet will tense noticeably. His testicles will retract, and his penis will stiffen to the ultimate. By then, his contractions have started, and his hips have begun thrusting. He might try to grind his pelvis into your face. This sounds pretty violent, but it could be more subtle, depending on the man.

If he grabs the back of your neck in an effort to place more pressure on his penis, or if he pulls your hair or ears, it is involuntary. If you are afraid or uncomfortable with this, gently remove his hands and place them on your shoulders or on his hips. If this excites you, then let him take control and hang on for the ride.

Once he has reached the point of no return, he will be bucking and grinding and grabbing. Do not stop what you are doing. Continue the same techniques, doing your best to maintain the same rhythm. You may have to hang onto his hips to control his movements, but for many guys, this just adds to the pleasure.

Where Does It Go?

In or Around Your Mouth. Hopefully, you have already decided where you want the come to go. Maybe you have even discussed it between yourselves. When you can tell he is about to ejaculate, or if he gives you the predetermined signal, pull back slightly. This will allow him to come on your tongue or your lips. Another option is to suck him deeply and let him come in the back of your throat. That way, you can swallow it if you so desire.

Other Body Parts. For something a little different, allow him to come on your breasts or belly or buttocks. This will require some prearranging on your part as well as his, but if it turns you on, it will be worth it.

Not in Your Mouth. If you don't want him to come in your mouth, or any other body part, be sure to have a towel nearby. When he comes, with his help, you can redirect it into the towel. If you forgot the towel, use the bed sheets.

A man's orgasm varies in length from five seconds to three minutes. Ejaculate is low in fat, calories, carbohydrates and high in quality protein. It also contains some zinc, calcium, magnesium, vitamins C and B-12, potassium, phosphorus and fructose. There is plenty of DNA in the mix, also. Now that forensic science is able to identify a person's DNA, many rapists are being caught. In the same way, many accused rapists, who were actually innocent, have been released from prison after serving many years. You can't get away from your own DNA.

8

For the Adventurous – Advanced Techniques

Fellatio in Our Everyday Sex Lives

Can participating in fellatio make a couple feel closer? It is possible. It depends on each of your attitudes toward the act. Do one or both of you feel it is evil or shameful? These ideas could interfere with any feelings of closeness you may be experiencing. The man who is receiving the blowjob may consider the act either a preliminary to, or a substitute for, regular intercourse. These attitudes and feelings must be addressed and dealt with if the experience of fellatio is a terrific one for you both.

Self-Pleasing

Masturbation

In order to enjoy the fellatio process, especially if the man is uptight or uncomfortable, a man must learn to participate in and enjoy masturbation. The majority of men in this country engage in masturbation to greater or lesser degrees depending on the guy's personal history and feelings.

If he believes that masturbation is distasteful or shameful, then it will require more than this book to change his mind. For the man who is willing, but naive or inexperienced, we do have a few suggestions. They are calculated to help him become familiar with, and learn to enjoy, the process of ministering to his own needs. Knowing how his body responds will help him when it is time to progress to fellatio.

1. Carve out a special time to be alone with yourself. Make sure that it is a relatively long stretch of time when you are not rushing between work and school and touch football. Bedtime is best, if you are alone. You can go to sleep right afterwards. (Is this where the habit of men falling immediately to sleep after sex originates?)

2. Begin slowly, with just the basics. Caress your genitals, including balls, penis and anus. At least try the anus, to see whether you like it or not. This knowledge will be helpful when you encounter sex with partners.

3. Work up to trying different techniques, just as you would with regular sex. Experiment with whatever toys strike your fancy.

4. Once you have mastered these techniques and have become familiar with your body and its reactions, you are ready to use them in lovemaking sessions with your significant other.

5. Masturbation can easily be overdone. It is fast, simple and noncommittal. These attributes can make it so intriguing that you may overindulge. Since it could make a man insensitive to another's mouth or vagina, it is best to err on the side of caution. If it happens to

you, stop completely for a period of time, especially if you anticipate engaging in fellatio.

Auto-Fellatio

The Questions. We are finally going to receive the answer to two world-shaking questions that have been plaguing man since the dawn of time: (1) if you could go down on yourself, would you, and (2) if you could go down on yourself, would you come in your own mouth?

The Practice. What is auto-fellatio? It is a man's ability to give himself a blowjob. He is able to take his penis into his own mouth and bring himself to orgasm.

Rarity. The practice of auto-fellatio is rarely seen even in pornography. It is also one of the few sex acts that is not mentioned in any law book—there is no law against it in any state. Besides, who is going to snitch on you (unless you decide to do it in tandem)?

According to Alfred Kinsey, between two and three men in every 1,000 are capable of going down on themselves. This meager statistic may be accounted for because the men who responded to Kinsey's survey were ashamed. They were reluctant to admit to performing an act that is most decidedly out of the usual male sexual experience.

While few human men are capable of auto-fellatio, our close relations, monkeys (Rhesus, macaques, mandrills and chimpanzees) do it quite handily. Mammals of other groups are also capable of self pleasuring.

Gary Griffin in *The Art of Auto-Fellatio* blames societal pressures and social taboos for its scarcity among humans. It appears as if many adolescents at least attempt it. Whatever the reason, most men discontinue their efforts long before adulthood.

Advanced Techniques

Deep Throat

Technique and Movie. The term "deep throat" refers to two things—a fellatio technique and the movie starring Linda Lovelace. When the movie first came out, it created quite a stir. I remember the first time I saw it. I was working at the county court house in Dallas, Texas, and the creators were being tried on obscenity charges. I sneaked into the courtroom and was able to view it with the jurors. There was a picture of me on the evening news coming out of the courtroom, smiling and waving at the cameras. Happily, my mother never saw that.

The popularity of this movie, and its representational technique, caused reverberations around the world. More particularly, male/female relationships were changed forever. After *Deep Throat*, every man thought his girlfriend should be able to do the same thing. Newsflash: just because porn stars can do certain death-defying acts doesn't mean the average person should attempt it. As with auto-fellatio, this technique requires some preparation, practice and patience. While it may seem like Nirvana to some men, others will tell you that they prefer other techniques. Therefore, saying that all men want or expect it is an inflation of the truth. As always, it depends on the guy.

Do not despair, however. It is easier to learn than auto-fellatio, and probably more people are physically capable of doing it. The keys are angle and position, breathing and rhythm—all working together to achieve the goal.

Where Throat and Mouth Meet. The first step to mastering this technique is a working knowledge of mouth and throat anatomy. We must learn where the mouth ends and the throat begins. The roof of the mouth is called the hard palate. As it continues to the back of the mouth, it becomes the soft palate. This is the area where the mouth ends and the throat begins.

Fellatio

Normally, when giving a blowjob, the penis does not extend past the mouth. Deep throating, however, requires swallowing between the throat and the openings of the windpipe and the esophagus, because that's how far your partner's penis will go.

The epiglottis is a crossing guard. Its purpose is to keep food and liquids from going down the larynx. Serving that purpose, it must decide whether to allow air into or out of the larynx, depending on messages it receives from the nerves. When it closes, air to the lungs is temporarily cut off. You stop breathing for a few moments. The same is true when you swallow the penis. You will be ceasing to breathe for a few moments, so timing is crucial.

The body's automatic response to the penis sliding down the throat is to attempt to expel it. As has been discussed previously, this involuntary nerve response is called gagging. The throat muscles constrict in an attempt to expel the object and prevent us from choking to death. This auto-response must be overcome in order to deep throat your lover's penis. Since it is a blowjob, the process of his penis going down your throat is going to be repeated over and over.

It is possible to learn not to gag when his penis tries to slip past your mouth and into your throat. I'm a little apprehensive about learning how not to gag. I mean, what if I am swallowing something else that I need to come back up, but I have been so efficient about overcoming my gagging sensation that I go ahead and swallow something like, say, one of the dog's bouncy balls? Okay, that's probably not going to happen, because you have to consciously overcome the gagging sensation. (Why do I have the dog's bouncy ball in my mouth in the first place? you might ask.) Presumably, you cannot learn to make it involuntary.

Here are a few tips to keep from gagging.

1. **Practice**. A dildo is a great penis substitute. If

you don't have one, buy one.
2. **Relax.** Stay relaxed all over, not just your head and mouth.
3. **Control.** Keep your hand on his penis in order to control his movements.
4. **Breathe.** Make sure you are continuing to breathe.
5. **Rest.** If you need to, take several breaks and rest or catch your breath.
6. **Angle.** Change the angle at which his penis enters your mouth.
7. **Distract.** Use your arousal to take your mind off the gagging effect.

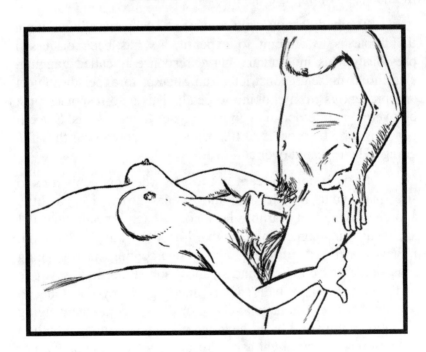

Figure 13: Deep Throat

Practice. Most sources recommend using a dildo to practice this technique, although penis-shaped vegetables, like

Fellatio

cucumbers and zucchinis, are also an option. Keep in mind that vegetables are slippery and could slip out of your hand while in your throat. Most of us wouldn't want to go to the emergency room with a cucumber stuck in our throats. On the other hand, you might already be dead since your airway is closed off, and who would call the ambulance anyway?

Use the base of the dildo to insert it into your mouth, giving yourself ample opportunity to get used to the way it feels. Push it a little farther back each time, until you begin to gag. Don't panic. Remember to exhale just before you put it in and inhale when you take it out. Practice until you feel confident enough to take on a real penis.

Position. The best position for deep throating is to lie on your back, thus elongating the neck and throat, while angling his penis into your throat. Some people hang their head over the side of the bed. Approaching the penis from above may prove easier with the angle excellent for deep penetration. Try this in conjunction with the 69 position.

Acupressure

Acupressure can bring something new to the table before a fellatio session. It is like a massage—and who doesn't love a massage—only much more highly concentrated. It will take some study and practice to find and manipulate the right spots, but for the person on the receiving end, it can release muscular tension and built-up toxins. The best way to do it is to hold the point for no longer than five minutes with the pads of your fingers. Be sure to avoid the protruding bones. You should have short fingernails, and the pressure you administer should be slow and direct. He should be breathing deeply as you press.

There are several specific points that will heighten the pleasure: (1) points at the top edge and center of the pubic bone; (2) the perineum; (3) inside the upper thigh; and (4) the base of the spine.

Changing Temperature/Taste of Mouth

Menthol or mint cough drops will cool your mouth and give it a tingly feel. Put them between your cheek and gums, not under your tongue. It might pop out. In the seventies, we were giving something called the "Binaca Blast." We sprayed the breath freshener Binaca into our mouths, and then went down on our man. He seemed to get a "blast" out of it. Then there was the "Crushed Ice Blowjob." Put the crushed ice in your mouth just ahead of his penis. A terrific and different sensation for his penis to experience.

Anal Insertions

Here's a warning: "Never insert anything into his anus that goes all the way in and disappears, even if your think it will dissolve." Okay, I guess that's just commonsense.

Masturbating During Fellatio

This is not exactly the most advanced suggestion, but it might enhance your fellatio session. While you are fellating your partner, try masturbating at the same time. Perhaps you can concentrate on two things at once, but I become a bit distracted when I pleasure myself. I have a tendency to forget about my partner. Perhaps you don't have that problem.

Adding a Friend or Two

Always discuss your feelings about group sex before you decide to add someone to your lovemaking sessions. You and your lover don't want to surprise each other with a guest unless you have cleared the way beforehand. It can get pretty sticky when one party has been surprised or coerced. Never do anything you don't feel comfortable doing, and never try to get someone else to do something they do not feel comfortable doing.

Public Fellatio

One of the advantages of fellatio is that it can be done practically anywhere. It can add to the sexual excitement if you decide to do it in a potentially public place. The fear of discovery can heighten the tension to the breaking point. Be careful when you are doing this, however. You don't want to be discovered by a child or a law enforcement officer. Make sure the spots you pick are secluded. Plan ahead and bring safe sex equipment with you.

9 Shake things up! New Positions

Versatility

Anywhere, Anytime

One of the finest aspects of fellatio is that it can be performed virtually anywhere and at any time. Even better, the recipient is most likely going to feel terrific regardless of how accomplished the giver might be or the position they use to perform the task. This creates a relaxed atmosphere (unless you are in a public place, as discussed in the previous chapter), which takes the performance pressure off of both parties.

Positions

Comfort

Worst Case Scenario. What is the worst possible thing that can happen in any sexual encounter? For some, it is that the man may last all night, or he might not ever ejaculate. No woman wants to be pounded away at all night. Regardless of how much fun it started out, after a couple of hours you are TIRED, you've climaxed about as much as you are going to, and you are ready to roll over and go to sleep. If the man has not orgasmed yet, he may want to continue until he does. What if he never does?

How much worse would this scenario be if you were giving the same man a blowjob? I would set a time limit on the encounter. If he isn't done by a certain period of time—however long it takes you to get a cramped tongue, an aching jaw and tight neck muscles—the party is over!

It may not take that long for one or all of these things to happen. If you're sure he's going to finish eventually, here are a few things you can do to make it less stressful and painful.

Comfortable Position. First and foremost, begin your encounter in a comfortable position, paying particular attention to your neck and shoulders. These are the two areas that are most affected. You should be able to maintain the position for at least 15 minutes or possibly longer. You may make minor adjustments as you progress. Hopefully, by the time you begin to cramp-up, he will be ready to explode. If not, set a time limit so you won't be totally stove-up the next day. It is okay to stop in the middle of things and change either your position or his. If you have to, ask him if he is close to coming. You should not feel bad about interrupting the flow in this situation. It might be the difference between having the event ruined for you and making it pleasant. If he's a nice guy, maybe he will give you a neck and back massage when you're done.

On Your Knees. Usually, you are going to be on your knees. You will most likely be on a bed, which would make a soft cushion for your knees. If the surface is hard, it can be quite painful for those with knee problems. If it is a long session, anyone may develop problems. Plan ahead, if you can, and have something soft, like a pillow or a blanket, nearby. If your knees just won't allow you to be on them for long, regardless, try crouching or squatting. Of course, if your knees are out of

Fellatio

shape, crouching or squatting may be as painful or more painful than your knees. If the bed or a pillow is out of the question, try reclining beside him.

Principal Position

Main Position. The most common or standard position for fellatio begins with the man lying on his back or leaning backward (usually propped against a headboard or wall). The person giving the blowjob kneels beside the man, approaching him in a perpendicular fashion. This angle allows the giver to employ a number of techniques. The entire genital area will be exposed, leaving it wide open to any ministrations the giver decides to provide.

The giver may also crawl between the man's knees and approach him from this angle. She may circle the body, stopping at any place she desires or that she believes will give her a comfortable approach and the man pleasure. Changing positions will help alleviate neck strain.

Classic Blowjob. Here are the steps for a classic blowjob:

Step 1: Touch the tips of your thumb and forefinger together, forming an "O" shape. Circle his penis with your fingers, then close the remainder of them around the shaft. It will look like a pig-in-a-blanket. Give his penis a squeeze.

Step 2: Glide your hand up and down his penis. Slip it into your mouth while still holding onto the shaft.

Step 3: Continue stroking with your hand as your mouth goes up and down on his penis. Be sure to stroke the same way, synchronizing your mouth and hand.

78   The Sensuous Couple's Guide to Seismic Oral Sex

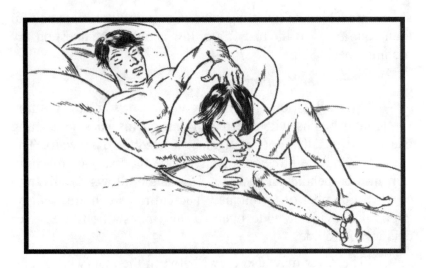

Figure 14: The Principal Position

Step 4: Continue this technique until you are ready to try something different, or until he is ready to come.

Position Variations

Variations on Main Position. If you have changed up the main position to place yourself between his knees, it would be fun to prop yourself up on your elbows. From this position, grab his buttocks or hips and place both his legs over your shoulders. This will delight him no end. Other choices—lightly push his knees against his chest; place his feet on your shoulders; sit on his legs (assuming you aren't an Amazon and he is a pigmy). If you decide to sit on his chest, try the variation of facing away from his head. He will appreciate the lovely view of your buttocks this gives him.

Lying. If he wants to lie down, you can lie next to him. If you want to lie down, he may sit on your chest or hover above your face. This provides maximum exposure of all body parts. He may thrust toward you or stay still, depending on your preference.

Fellatio

You may lie on your back with your head hanging off the edge of the bed. This will stretch your throat and make it more open, thus reducing the gag factor. As discussed earlier, this is the best position if you plan to deep throat. He will be standing over you doing the thrusting, which may place you in a vulnerable position. However, your hands will be free, and you can use them to control the thrusting if it becomes necessary.

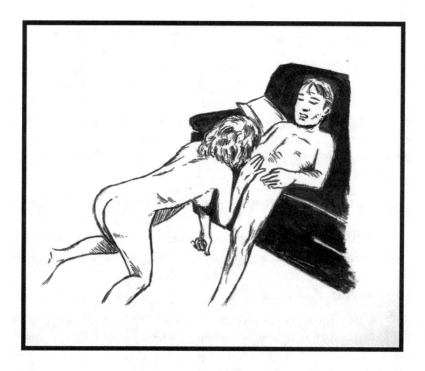

Figure 15: Seated Position

Seated. If he would rather be seated than lying down, have him sit on the edge of a bed, chair or table. You will then kneel in front of him to do your business. If you want to be the one seated, take a chair and have him stand over you.

Tea Bagging. This technique entails taking one or both of his balls completely into your mouth. Suck lightly or hum while your mouth is full of his testicles.

Hands and Knees. This position requires a flexible penis (and possibly a long one). Have him bend over, while you get on all fours behind him. Suck his penis, stroke his perineum, lick his balls or rim his anus, if you both have agreed that it would give you pleasure. All these parts are available from the doggie position.

Anal Penetration

Go Slowly. Although a guy may love for you to play around his anus, he may draw the line at actual penetration. Be sure to check ahead to make sure it is okay. You might want to begin very slowly and assess his reactions as you advance. If he acts the least bit squeamish, then you should stop what you are doing immediately. In other words, pay attention and use plenty of lubricant.

Anus Unlubricated. Unlike the mouth, the vagina or the penis, the anus does not produce its own lubricant. The skin around the opening is thin and sensitive. This characteristic makes playing with the area pleasurable, but it can also cause pain. Your man may come just by having his anus touched; however, this is exceptionally rare.

Beginning Technique. The first step in anal penetration is cleanliness. Make sure your hands are washed and your nails are smoothly trimmed. After everything that you are doing to him has turned him on sufficiently, begin to press and squeeze his buttocks. Lightly tease your fingers around his anal opening, moving them in a circular motion. If you have not done so before, lubricate a finger and slowly begin to press it into the anal opening. Slide the finger up to the first joint. Do not go any further until you have given him time to get used to the feeling. Take several breaths, perhaps slowly turn your finger around and feel his muscles contract. Do not move the finger further inside until his muscles have relaxed. Then, continue to slide it

Fellatio

in a bit more at a time. Mimic intercourse by making a small in-and-out motion with your finger, proceeding very gently. Before long, he will become accustomed to the feeling of something inside him.

Prostate Stimulation. Once you have him used to finger stimulation, you can now attempt to find his prostate from the inside. It sits just below the bladder, and the penis is more or less anchored to it. There is a nerve bundle that is located just beneath the prostate, which will create a sensation in the penis if it is stimulated internally. The prostate can be the size of a small chestnut or large walnut. It swells and becomes firm when the man is aroused. This should help you locate it.

Once you have your finger on the right spot, curve it slightly toward the front of the man's body. Make a come-hither motion, but do it carefully. The prostate is a delicate organ. The movement of your finger may create a peeing sensation, which your man may not like. Unconsciously, he may even leak a little. If he does like it, however, and is stimulated to orgasm, he will have a powerful and intense experience.

Rimming

"Rimming" is using your tongue to stimulate his anus. This is a pretty advanced technique. The giver and/or the receiver may find it abhorrent. If you have discussed it beforehand, and you both are game, then go for it. Here are a few ways to get into it: kiss the opening of the anus until you are ready to use your tongue; press your tongue flat against the anus and lick up and down; use the tip or your tongue to lick a ring around the rim, then carefully insert the tip into the anal opening.

Dart your tongue in and out. If you moan, it will simulate a vibrator, and get him more excited. When you sense that he is about to come, use your hand to finish the job. He will be yours for life.

82   The Sensuous Couple's Guide to Seismic Oral Sex

Sixty-Nine (69) is when both parties are giving oral sex to their partners at *the same time. If you are pleasuring your guy with fellatio, it* would be wonderful if he reciprocated. This can be accomplished with him on his hands and knees over you, or with you on top, hands and knees over him, or both of you lying on your sides. Both of you can use the techniques you have learned in this book.

It should be an unbelievably exhilarating experience!

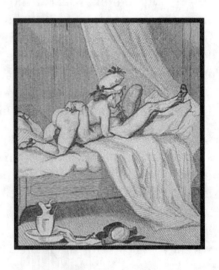

Figure 16: Félicien Rops Engraving illustrating the sex position "69". Published in 1865, France

10 Fantasies and Practices

Fantasies

Fantasizing Not Cheating

Fantasizing does not necessarily mean that you want to act on the fantasy. If you are dreaming about a movie star while having sex with your partner, you should not feel guilty, or feel as if you are cheating. This has probably been said a thousand times and in every sex instruction or information book written, but some are still not getting the message. Remember, they are called "fantasies" because they are not real life.

Gender Playing

You may have a fantasy of playing the part of the opposite gender. If you are a female, you might dream of buckling up a strap-on and putting it to your male partner in the rear. Or you may want to give it to your female partner in the vagina. If you are a male, you might wonder about the feeling of a penis inside you, but you don't want another man. If you and the female with the strap-on get together, it will be a perfect union of consenting, gender-swapping adults.

Practices

Penis Enlargement

Pills. Have you seen the advertisements about how happy Dick and his spouse are because Dick used an all-natural penis enhancement supplement? Do not fall for it. There is no pill presently on the market that can make your penis larger. Period.

Vacuum Pumps. These may work temporarily, but must be used properly. Otherwise, they can cause irreversible damage. My best friend in high school dated a man who had cancer. He was forced to use a pump because it was the only way he could sustain an erection. She liked it—sex-on-demand, not a bad option. Another caution is that they will create a large erection, but it is a soft one, which may not be all that useful. Didn't seem to bother my high school friend, though, because sex was slower and closer to her natural rhythm.

Implants. Surgery is required in order to place silicone implants inside the penis. Be aware that surgery cuts through nerves, fibers and erectile tissue—all necessary items when an erection and sexual enjoyment are desired. Implants may become infected and have to be replaced. In addition, they can look and feel lumpy.

In other words, forget about it. As we noted earlier, most penises enlarge to close to the same size when they become erect, so artificial enlargement is normally unnecessary.

Pleasure and Pain

Closely Related. We all know that pleasure can become pain and vice versa. Sometimes, when pleasure is too intense, it can be painful. When pain is not too intense, it can be pleasurable. For example, when all the feel-good drugs produced by our bodies during sex kick in, we could introduce a little pain into the mix. It might feel like pleasure. As always, such a thing needs to be discussed beforehand with your partner. There are an array of techniques and toys that would enhance the sexual experience with a little or a lot of pain, depending on your bent.

Here are a few that do not include sex toys, as they will be covered in the next chapter:

1. Spank his thighs or butt cheeks with the flat of your hand. (Never spank or slap his testicles, or you will have him slapping you right back.)
2. Nibble or bite his butt, stomach or nipples. His nipples will most likely be very sensitive and tender right before orgasm, which would be a good time to do this. Not too hard though, unless he likes it hard.
3. Scratch him with your fingernails. Remember all the movies you've seen where one partner wakes up after a night of torrid sex with deep scratch marks on his or her back? (Or maybe that was just in *Rosemary's Baby*, when she had sex with the devil.)
4. Tickle him, if he can stand it and wants you to.
5. Very lightly scrape his penis with your teeth.

This should feel only slightly painful, not extremely. Most people do not tolerate extreme pain well. This is called "sadomasochism," (see **Glossary**) and is enjoyed by a minority. We will discuss some aspects of sadomasochism in the next chapter.

11 Devices and Toys

Pain as Pleasure

While it is a common conception that pain and pleasure are closely related, actually wanting to feel pain in any form whatsoever is a matter of choice. This would not be my personal choice, although I do enjoy having my nipples lightly bitten as sexual foreplay. Once, a guy spanked me on the butt, and I got so tickled I could barely continue the session. I just couldn't take it seriously enough for it to be erotic. There are many people, however, who find the line between pleasure and pain to be so thin as to be easily crossed over. The following toys and devices are for them. These devises are highly varied in nature, and will accomplish any pain/pleasure goal the participants might have set.

As we have stated many times before, communication with the other person is of utmost importance, especially in this area of administering pain. The parties should have selected a word the receiving party can say that curtails the action immediately. The word should be agreed upon beforehand. When the receiver utters it, the giver must be prepared to completely stop whatever they are doing.

Shopping for Sex Toys

Know what you want, and go to the best place you can find to get it. If you don't have any high-class places in your city (see ***Bibliography*** for recommendations), then use the Internet or phone order. On the Internet, you won't have as much information as you can get from shops and catalogs. If you have a catalog, you can ask questions when you phone in your order.

Clamps and Clips

Application. Clamps and clips can be applied to many body parts, including the nipples, penis and testicles. To attach, merely pinch up a piece of skin, squeeze the clip open, place over skin and let the clip go. This type of pain is usually low-level, but continuous. Some clips and clamps provide a way to vary its tightness. Once the clamp has been in place for a period of time, quickly unclip it. The blood supply, which has heretofore been cut off, will rush back to the clipped area with a vengeance. In this situation, the pain can be powerful, which can cause intense pleasure for some.

Where to Buy. Buy these devices at S&M shops or stationery stores. If you work in an office, you can steal them from your employer. I find that the medium-sized black ones have different spring pressures: some are easily opened; others are very tight. You can pick the tension that best suits your needs.

CBT

Anytime the word "torture" enters into the picture, most of us are going to opt out of whatever might be in store. However, we must remember that one man's Spanish Inquisition is another man's liberation army. Hence, we are learning about "CBT" or "cock and ball torture."

As we have learned, a man's genital area is highly sensitive and contains countless nerves. For this reason, it is the go-to area when desiring to administer pleasurable pain.

Floggers. Floggers are the medium used to torture his genitals. They come in small, medium and large, just like penis sizes. Each size should be used for a different purpose. His balls are the most sensitive area of a man's genitals. Since you don't want to injure them, use the small flogger on his testicles. Use medium-sized floggers on his penis, unless he is less sensitive to pain than most. In that case, use a large flogger. It is best to begin small and work up, depending on his reaction. Watch how he reacts and keep up the communication. You don't want it to be so painful that he is not enjoying it.

Cock Rings. These devises are not necessarily made for pain. Their purpose is to restrict blood flow. By steadily squeezing the penis and the testicles, they increase the intensity of pleasure and extend the length of his erection. (Not the length of his penis, but how long his erection lasts.) Cock rings can be made of various materials. They come in leather, plastic and rubber. While they are normally not meant to inflict pain, there are some that will. These can be found in specialty stores. They are constructed in such a manner that fishing weights and leashes can be added.

Ball Devises. The testicles are the most sensitive part of the man's genitalia, so several devises are made to administer pleasurable pain to them. These concoctions include stretchers, vises, stocks and separators, etc. There are too many to mention, so do some research to locate what you think will work best for your situation.

Other Devices

Pinwheel. The pinwheel is used by physicians to determine a person's nerve response. A stainless steel rolling wheel is attached to an eight-inch handle. The pin-prick edge of the rolling wheel is rolled over the skin. During a sexual encounter, this device can be rolled across any part of the receiver's body. Because of its ability to administer great pain, avoid the most sensitive areas, such as the penis, testicles and anus. It can prick the skin deeply, so use it lightly over the areas you do pick.

Anal. Make sure your anal toys have long handles and flared bases so that you don't lose them inside. Butt plugs are made to be left inside the anus until ejaculation. They also come in a vibrating variety. Butt beads need to be lubricated before insertion. Pull them out when he begins to orgasm. Finally, try the vibrating anal-T, which serves to vibrate his prostate and bring him ecstatically to orgasm.

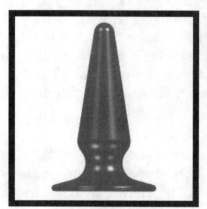

Figure 17: Butt Plug

Pleasure without Pain

Tie Me Up, Tie Me Down

Restraints. You won't have to spend much money for this little trick. In fact, you probably have a piece of rope already lying around the house. If you are with someone who enjoys the feeling of being completely at your mercy, this may be the proper technique. It requires a measure of trust, just as many of these suggestions do. If you want to go to the store, buy some handcuffs to make your partner feel even more helpless. Get several interchangeable keys, and don't lose them.

Blindfolds. Blindfolds are as cost-effective as restraints. When you tie your Hermes (or Wal-Mart) scarf around your guy's eyes, he can surrender to your attentions without any distractions. If you want a blindfold that fits better than whatever you drug out of the closet, you may buy them specifically created for sexual encounters. These fit better, are more comfortable, and stay put longer than homemade blindfolds. A specialty item is not necessary, however, so don't let it prevent an impromptu performance.

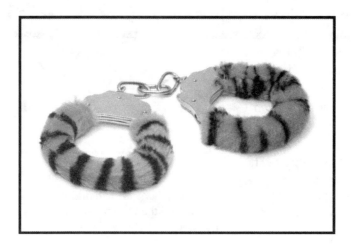

Figure 18: Fun Furry Handcuffs

The Wonderful World of Strap-Ons

What is a Strap-On? A strap-on is a harness with a dildo attached meant to emulate a penis. It enables the person (probably a woman, since she doesn't have a penis) wearing it to do the same things to a man (or another woman) that a man could do (except come). It is commonly associated with lesbian couples, but recent information indicates that gay men and heterosexual couples are buying them in droves.

Heterosexual Couples. Perhaps the male partner of a heterosexual couple suffers from erectile dysfunction. He can still pleasure his woman the way he normally would by using a strap-on. If a non-gay man desires to experience the feeling of penetration, then his female partner can employ a strap-on to give him an erotic experience he is unlikely to experience otherwise. Just the sight of a woman wearing a dildo can be a mind-blowing experience for some men. It can be used during a roll swapping session.

Strap-Ons and Fellatio. Believe it or not, it has been suggested that going down on a dildo is a sexual encounter some people can't resist. Obviously, it is for viewing purposes only. The dildo is not going to come. That would be an interesting invention, one I believe is possible.

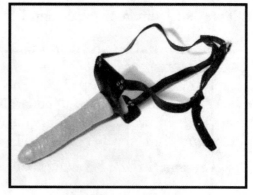

Figure 19: Strap-on

Two - strap harness with dildo; the outer strap goes around the wearer's waist, while the inner strap goes between his/her legs.

After all, remember the "Betsy Wetsy" doll? The man allegedly should become excited merely by watching you go down on a penis, whether it is his real one or not. Men are mostly visual, so use lots of visual techniques and your hands to enhance the show. Try using the techniques and tricks we have introduced to you just as if you were ravishing a real penis.

Buying Tips. Be sure to buy the harness and the dildo as separate units, but make sure the dildo is specifically made for a harness. Single units are usually not as good as separate parts. Final tip: buy these products from a reputable boutique, particularly one that caters to women. You will get a better product.

Vibrators and Dildos

Vibrators. The pulsation from vibrators can be intense, especially on the head of his penis. Some men enjoy the feeling, but prefer you to avoid more sensitive areas. Some areas that

Fellatio

would be good candidates for vibration are: beneath the head of the penis, the underside of the shaft, the testicles (but take it easy), perineum and anus. Small vibrators that can be worn on the end of your finger are available. They can be used to give great pleasure to the other person's anus. Please do not insert them into the anus, however, or anywhere else! They could come off your finger and get lost up his butt. As we have said before, and it bears repeating, anything that gets inserted into the anus must have a flared base. This precaution is meant to prevent the device from slipping all the way inside and becoming irretrievable. Neither of you want to be checking in at the emergency room with that particular problem.

Strap-Ons. We have already discussed strap-ons, which can have various speed and motion selections. If you insist on the very best, then buy silicone. It is excellent, but expensive. Less expensive, but still quite good, is hard plastic. Never use anything that is porous. It could retain moisture and attract bacteria and other undesirable things. Throw it away, or use a condom when using it.

Dildos. Dildos come in all shapes, sizes, colors and materials. Some even come with their own testicles. They are specifically made for insertion and do not vibrate.

Books and Magazines

We are living in the age of information. If you can read, you can become an expert on any subject. Sex instruction and information are no different.

Books. Books are one of the best tools you can utilize when beginning your fellatio career (or any other sexual act you are new to). No other source has as much variety or as detailed information. Both parties in a relationship can use books to enhance their sexual encounters.

Black Lace, a women's anthology publisher, produces books that focus on heterosexuality. Although their literature does contain homosexual characters, the thrust (no pun intended) is male/female sex. The fellatio in these series of books is reportedly great.

Buy an instruction manual on sex the same way you buy a book about decorating or cooking. If the cover appeals to you, pick up the book and read the back cover. Open it and scan the table of contents. Pick out a subject you are interested in, go to that page and read a few paragraphs. See if the tone and writing are on your desired level. Is there enough detail? Too much? Illustrations? If it appears to be repetitious of information you already have, look for something else. Focus on books that expand your knowledge.

Magazines. What are the magazines that we think of when we think about sex? *Playboy? Hustler?* Others that are perhaps more hard core? Most of these magazines cater to men or to a specific variation, i.e., gay porn. With the exception of *Playgirl*, very few appeal specifically to women.

Videos

Videos as Sex Toys. Pornographic videos may be the best sex toys around. They offer something books cannot—moving imagery. The illusion (or reality) that the sex act is occurring can be very stimulating. If you are performing fellatio, a good video will do much of the work for you. Videos come in three types: soft core, hard core and instructional.

Rentals and Purchases. Many people would not be caught dead in the adult section of a video store. Others camp out there. Most are in the middle. We like an occasional adult video to enhance our sex lives, but we feel a wee bit sleazy and self-conscious lurking in the adult section.

Overcoming this reluctance is apparently not too difficult. Millions of people rent adult movies every year. It must be men, you might think, and gay men at that. Women and couples are jumping onto the porno bandwagon. They are renting and buying sex tapes in greater numbers than ever before.

Fellatio

Women and Imagery. A nonsensical myth has been perpetuated for years—all my life, actually—that women do not respond to visual imagery. Few sex videos are made for women because of this ridiculous myth. Nothing could be farther from the truth. While they may not admit it, a study in Amsterdam in 1994 proved that women's bodies respond involuntarily to sexually stimulating images. Their genitals filled with blood, a symptom of being aroused, in spite of what they were admitting to verbally.

Lower Expectations. Like on-line dating (or any dating, for that matter), it is better to lower your expectations when shopping for an adult film. You are not going to get the same quality as Hollywood mainstream movies. Not even as good as independent films. They are shot on a budget (a very small one, usually), and the sets, lights and cameras are inexpensive and simple. And the acting? What acting? Keep the remote control nearby. You can cut to the chase (which usually doesn't take too long anyway) if it gets too boring.

Wide Appeal. Most adult videos follow the same standards and formulas. If you have ever seen a soft core porno video on cable TV, you will see that there are certain scenes, positions and couplings that are mandatory. All porno videos have them. The actors and actresses have shaved genitals. The women's breasts are large. In hard core porn, the men's penises are usually larger than average.

In hard core porn, as a rule, the men pull out before ejaculation. They come somewhere on the other person, like their face, breasts or butts. No one seems to care if the woman ejaculates. If it can't be seen, it must not be important, right? That attitude, however, is gradually changing. The Showtime original series, "Family Business," features Seymour Butts. He is a sometime porno-actor who is making a female ejaculation film. His female subject ejaculates much like a man. At one point, she spurts onto the camera. That's one place the actor or actress isn't supposed to ejaculate.

Personal Desires. Before venturing into the video store for the first time, make sure you have a good idea what you are looking for. What are your expectations? What do you want to see? What do you not want to see? Making a list of your likes and dislikes before picking out the movie will be helpful. Check out the review and ratings. Consult with your partner if you are planning on letting them in on the action. Want a little more subtlety and class than what you get from the average video? Try viewing a movie directed by a female. Remember, however, that porno is never really what you would call "subtle."

Instructional. Typical porno videos are not designed to be instructional materials. They are created strictly for looks. In other words, they are not showing you the most comfortable or efficient positions. They are showing you the ones that look best from the camera's point of view.

Buy one that is specifically instructional, especially if you are looking to learn fellatio techniques. Be forewarned that these videos all appear to have originated in the eighties. There is a fireplace, furry rug and fluffy hair. The action is narrated by talking heads who claim to be experts. This tends to come off rather creepy as opposed to professional, but there are a few exceptions. These exceptions are created by mainstream adult film stars or independents produced by sex toy companies, individuals or sex organizations.

Lubricants

General. If you haven't been to the local sex shop, you can use saliva as a lubricant. If you prefer something a little more sophisticated, then go for a water-based lubricant. They are the best and the safest, as oil-based will melt latex. Make sure, if you are using it for vaginal insertion, that it is FDA-approved for vaginal use. Colorless formulas will wash out of fabric. If you are not going to use it vaginally with a condom, then try silicone. It is more slippery, doesn't dry out and is recommended for anal play. Before using the lubricant, rub it around in the palm of your hands until the friction heats it up. This will feel sublime against skin.

Rimming. Some people think flavored lubricants taste really badly, but I'm wondering . . . do they taste any worse than somebody's asshole? Do not buy lubricant that is made specifically for anal sex. They contain numbing agents, which is the last thing you want. These lubricants will not only numb the anus, they will numb your tongue as well. If you are doing anal penetration properly, it should not hurt. And flavored lubricants are not going to make an act you find abhorrent any less so.

Edible. Lubricants can be either water-based or oil based. The edible ones contain oil, which means they melt latex. So, if you are planning on having penetrative sex later, use the water-based. Other oily items that are often used in sex, such as whipped cream and chocolate topping, should also be avoided if you are using a latex condom. In addition, because of their high sugar content, they may cause yeast infections.

12 Believe It or Not

Facts

Penis

Believe It or Not. Have you ever had a guy tell you that he "hangs right" or "hangs left"? It's true; his penis is either "left-handed" or "right handed." The first time a man told me that, I thought he was kidding. He told me, and I don't know if this is true or not, that they made suit pants fuller on one side or the other, depending on which way his penis hung. Your guy's penis is larger than a mountain gorilla's member. Proportionally speaking, that is, compared to his body size. An ejaculation can reach up to 28 miles per hour, but don't ask me how they measured this. I'm thinking about those machines that they use to measure fast balls in baseball.

Testicles

These little beauties produce somewhere between 200,000,000 and 600,000,000 sperm per ejaculation. They hang outside the body, rather than inside, because it's cooler out there. They maintain a temperature perfect for creating those millions of sperm. Why is one lower than the other? To keep them from bumping into each other when the man walks or crosses his legs. The human body is a wondrous thing.

Myths of Male Sexuality

Oversimplification

Men and Pleasure. Isn't a man's sexuality a simple thing, like a faucet? You turn it on, the water comes out, and you are done. Nothing to it, right? Their genitalia is so upfront and obvious, we tend to think it is really that simple. Like a faucet, we forget the complex mechanism that keeps it running. Never forget that men are all different, even if their plumbing is basically the same. Women's magazines give us little insight into how men enjoy sex. It is a complicated issue that cannot be summed up in articles oversimplifying what men want, and what you can do to give it to them.

Perpetrators of Stereotype. Urban legend dictates that a blowjob is all a man really wants, and the media perpetuates this myth. If you give him one, or the promise of one, he is a wind-up doll who will respond to anyone, anytime, and immediately. Every female I know also perpetuates this myth. Common consensus says that a man can be led around by his penis. It is the key whereby the wind-up doll is turned on. Men have no needs other than the obvious.

If you are guilty of perpetuating this attitude, you are missing out on a great opportunity to understand your man's needs and wants on a much deeper level. If you are willing to take the time and effort to do this, if you really care about him, it will deepen the bond between you.

Problems

Impotency

Universal. Every man at one time in his life has been unable to produce or maintain an erection. There are myriad reasons for this phenomenon. When it happens, the man's partner should not show their frustration. The best advice I ever heard was to just ignore it. Don't point it out or make fun. Don't even try to discuss it with him in a sympathetic way. Just pretend it didn't happen. It is normally situational rather than chronic. If it is chronic, it may be due to illness or psychological reasons. In this situation, help should be sought.

Drugs. There are several pills on the market that are supposed to fix the problem of impotence. Be forewarned, however, that these are not aphrodisiacs. The man must be aroused before they will work. If he has psychological problems, they won't be of any help. They only work if the problem is physiological.

A drug called Levitra seems to give men the best performance, according to researchers Even though Cialis's effects may last longer, patients appeared to prefer the quick onset of action of Levitra. It was reliable and produced a satisfactorily hard erection. Both drugs proved effective, as did the third choice, Viagra. They produced a significant improvement in erections for vaginal penetration and completion of intercourse. The effect of these drugs is cumulative. The longer you take them, the more effective they become. Researchers recommended that a man stay on Viagra if it works well for him, and he has one or two sexual episodes a month. Try Levitra if you don't have sex frequently, are diabetic, or have had prostrate surgery. Cialis is good for sexually active males and is the most cost-effective. A new drug called Uprima is being tested. It acts in a different manner than Viagra and works faster. It is dissolved under the tongue, causing it to enter the blood stream faster.

Be sure to check with your physician and do your

research when electing to take any type of drug. All drugs have side effects, and impotency drugs have been discouraged for men who take blood pressure lowering medications. Be sure to stay away from alcohol when taking these drugs.

Dependable Erections. A man should see a doctor for any physical or psychological reason for not having dependable erections. Aside from this, the best way to improve the quality of erections is to practice, practice, practice. Regular stimulation and regular sex, either with yourself or a partner, will keep the genitals oxygenated and exercised. The penis is a muscle, and it requires oxygen and exercise to keep it strong. Don't overdo it though. See why in the next paragraph.

Inability to Ejaculate

Reasons. Even if a man is able to maintain an erection, he may not be able to ejaculate. One of the main reasons a man may fail to ejaculate is because he masturbates frequently or has sex very often with a partner. Also, he may ejaculate more than once or twice with a partner. While we recommend regular sex, don't overdo it. Some people require more sex than others. Each individual will have to measure for themselves what is the proper amount.

Another reason a man might not be able to ejaculate is alcohol. Excessive amounts of alcohol can lead to both the inability to ejaculate and the inability to maintain or achieve an erection.

There are medical conditions that may cause the inability to ejaculate, such as street or prescription drugs, or a condition called retrograde ejaculation.

Retrograde Ejaculation. Men who have a spinal cord injury or prostate or bladder surgery may have this problem. When a man is about to ejaculate, the opening between the bladder and the urethra closes, and the ejaculate expels normally. If, for whatever reason, this valve does not close, the fluid goes into the bladder rather than coming out the penis.

Fellatio

This is not usually painful. If it is, a physician should be consulted.

Disabilities

Injuries. If you are dealing with a man with an injury or disability, fellatio may be the answer. Most injuries do not interfere with a man's lust. Even if his leg is broken, he still wants to make love or have it made to him. Back strains, casts and the like can be dealt with using pillows and other devices. Use your imagination to come up with ways calculated to make the injured man more relaxed and at ease with sex.

Illness. A paralyzed man still has possession of many of his faculties. He can still see, smell and hear. He may have the same feelings he had before, but may not be able to show them as in the past. ADD sufferers and others may be inhibited by drugs. Fellatio may be just the right technique to administer to these impaired men.

Communication. In situations such as injuries and illness, communication is vital. You must express to each other what you desire, and what you are willing and able to perform. Once you are comfortable talking about his needs (and yours), then progress to the next step. Try to remain open minded and maintain a playful attitude. You will amaze yourself at the myriad techniques the two of you come up with. Cooperation will lead to mutual pleasure.

13 Safe Oral Sex

There are two periods in modern sexual history: Pre-HIV and Post-HIV. If you were sexually active pre-HIV, you didn't have very much to worry about, except syphilis (rare and easily curable with penicillin), gonorrhea and crabs. If you were pre-pill, you had to worry about getting pregnant.

Times have changed. Boy, have they changed! Before, you were pretty sure if you had sex you probably weren't going to die. That is no longer true. The risks of contracting a fatal disease from sex is very high. It can happen not only with a stranger, but with someone who is quite close to you. You must protect yourself at all times.

At the very least, USE A CONDOM! Please use a latex barrier for all sexual activities that entail the passing of fluid between two people. Unfortunately, in this dangerous world, there are many people who do not do this, and they are putting their lives at risk every time. One friend contracted Hepatitis C. She is undergoing Interferon therapy, and it is not fun. Plus, there are no guarantees that it will free her of the disease.

Risks of Unprotected Fellatio

Sexually Transmitted Diseases

STDs. You are a man, and a lovely woman has placed you on your back, removed your briefs and is ready to go down on you. You are in sexual ecstasy and are not thinking about anything, except the pleasure you are about to receive. All you have to do now is just lay back, relax and enjoy. Right?

Wrong! Fellatio is a two person sex act, and you are in some danger of sexually transmitted diseases ("STDs"), just as you would be if you were having intercourse. While the risk may not be as high as penis/vaginal or penis/anus sex, it is still very real. If the man ejaculates, the risk is moderate; if the man does not ejaculate, the risk is low. But it is still a risk.

Fellatio and STDs. Both viral and bacterial STDs may be transmitted during fellatio. The person who is giving and the person who is receiving are both at risk if the man is not wearing a condom. Some of the myriad diseases that can be transmitted by unprotected sex are HIV, hepatitis B and C, herpes, syphilis, gonorrhea, HPV (human papillomavirus–genital warts), etc.

Rimming and STDs. Rimming, like fellatio, can be highly pleasurable to those who are open to the technique. Like fellatio, however, it is not safe. It is even less safe than fellatio, and it is highly recommended that it not be performed without a barrier.

Warnings and Suggestions

Warnings

Dental Work. Don't go to the dentist before you engage in oral sex. Sores and cuts in the mouth are just passageways for STDs. Some experts recommend to not even brush or floss, as these activities produce tiny cuts on the gums. Instead of not brushing or flossing before a hot date, perhaps you should put off the fellatio until the next morning. Do it before you get up and brush your teeth.

Gloves. Your lips, tongue and mouth are not the only body parts you use when you perform fellatio. Your hands are employed as much or more than the others. For this reason, we advise putting on latex gloves before you handle a stranger's penis, balls or anus.

Suggestions

Tests. Some precautions can be bypassed if you have established a relationship with one person. Both of you must be tested for all STDs before these precautions are thrown out the window. I recommend going to a clinic at the same time, and showing each other your test results. From this point you can make an agreement to (1) remain monogamous, (2) only have unprotected sex with each other and use barriers with all others. I would recommend commencing an investigative search on the other party. This can be done through the internet by a company who specializes in this type of thing. This may sound invasive, but we are talking about your life here.

Sexual History. Before you put something in your mouth, it is better to know where it's been first. True, there are all kinds of hustlers and unethical people out there, and no guarantees that the person is telling you the truth. Consequently, it is better to use barriers for all sexual activities for several months. After that, have your blood tests. If you are both negative, you could proceed with suggestions (1) or (2) above. Take your time. Get to know the person. If you are the least bit suspicious, or even if you are not, have them checked out by a private investigator.

Safety is Sexy. It sounds as if having sex these days may be more trouble than it is worth. We are forced to suit up as if we were going into a radiation-contamination area. We zip ourselves into germ-proof suits, pull out our air-filtering headgear, and slip on our total-coverage gloves and shoes. It appears as if we are gearing up for biological warfare rather than preparing to give sexual pleasure to another anticipating adult.

We ARE protecting ourselves from environmental biohazards. If we want to save our lives, we must be willing to do what it takes. What we need to change is our attitude. Instead of grumbling about the extra expense, the dulling of sensual pleasure or the ridiculous inconvenience, why not make these disease barriers part of our fantasies? Make learning to use them an amusing adventure. Accept them with open arms and use our imaginations and senses of humor to create fun, unusual and exciting sexual experiences. My mind is creating all sorts of scenarios even as I write this. I'll bet your mind can do the same.

Condoms and Other Protections

Condoms

Rules of Use. Condoms should be used for all sexual activities, whether vaginal, oral or anal. Without exception, they should be used every time you participate in these activities. Use them properly as well. Do not use them past their expiration date and never use a sexual barrier a second time. Please refrain from getting inebriated to assure that you put the condom (or other barrier) on correctly.

Installation Instructions. Condoms may be put on either manually or orally.

Fellatio

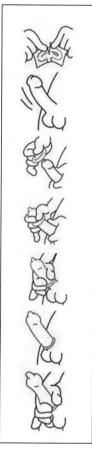

Manual. Here are the instructions for putting on a condom before intercourse or fellatio:

1. Carefully open the package. Do not use your teeth or a sharp object to avoid ripping, cutting or tearing the condom. Do not unroll it.
2. The penis should be hard before the condom is applied. The uncircumcised man should pull back his foreskin. Place the condom on the end (head) of the penis, being careful to put it on correctly. If it is put on backwards, it must be removed and discarded. Open a new one, and start from the beginning.
3. Squeeze the air out of the condom by pinching the tip between your thumb and index finger. Roll the condom onto the penis. It should reach all the way to the base. No space should be left at the tip. The condom should not be broken or compromised in any way.

Figure 20: Manual Installation

Oral. Here are the instructions for putting on a condom with your teeth:

1. Use an unlubricated condom because lubricated ones will taste bad.
2. Once you have removed the packaging, place the unfolded condom in your mouth. Position it on the inside of your cheek, between your teeth, with the tip pointing inward. Be careful not to bite the condom.

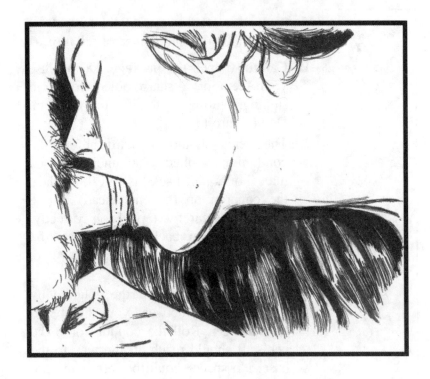

Figure 21: Putting a Condom on With Your Mouth

3. Work it over to the front of your mouth. Avoid using your teeth as much as possible. Put your mouth on the penis and begin rolling the condom down with your lips, tongue and teeth. Go gently in order to avoid tearing the condom.

4. Once the condom reaches the base of the penis, you are done.

You are now ready to insert the penis for intercourse or for fellatio.

Fellatio

Here are the instructions for removing the condom after intercourse or fellatio:

1. Hold onto the condom at the base of the penis. Remove it from the vagina or mouth before the penis becomes soft.
2. Slide the condom off the penis, holding it in such a way to avoid spilling the semen inside.
3. Dispose of the used condom in the trash receptacle. Do not flush it down the toilet. It will stop up the sewer system.

Unflavored. Here are a few recommendations for condoms to use when engaging in fellatio.

- Durex Clear Unlubricated—a basic, straightforward condom.
- Trojan Enz—cream-colored, reservoir tip, average everything.
- Ria colored condoms—comes in variety of colors and are fun.
- Trojan Non Lube—favorite of fellatio aficionados; plain rounded end; no reservoir tip; longer than average.

Flavored. Here are a few recommendations for flavored condoms:

- Durex Flavored.
- Kiss of Mint (Lifestyles).
- Trustex Flavored.

Nonlatex. Here are a few recommendations for nonlatex condoms:

- Avanti Polyurethane—better than latex because twice as thin and strong; preferred because have no taste.

- Trojan Supra—thin, soft in texture; hypoallergenic; no taste or smell.

Other Forms of Protection

There are myriad other protections for sexual activities. A few of them are: gloves, finger cots, dental dams and plastic wraps. Decide which practices you want to engage in, study what protection is available, and use them accordingly. But whatever you do, use them!

14 Common & Uncommon Questions

Question: Do Altoids Breath Mints really create an astounding blowjob?

This particular idea became popular as an email widely circulated since 1997. Like all such emails, it attests to the truth of its assertions. If a woman has a box of Altoids on their desk, they are supposed to be part of the "Secret Blowjob Goddess Society." This so-called society got its start when a woman, who was a smoker, chewed several of the mints in order to freshen her breath before giving her latest beau a blowjob. Even after she broke up with him, he was exclaiming about the merits of her technique, and that he had never experienced anything like it. After thinking about what she had done to him that was different from her earlier encounters, she gave credit for the fabulousness of her blowjob to the Altoids.

Being a generous woman, she allegedly passed this information on to other women and the society was born. Now, every single woman and every married man is on a rampage to buy Altoids. If this story is true, don't we wish we had invested in Altoid stocks?

For the record, Altoids do leave a lasting tingle which may or may not be stronger than other breath mints. This is based strictly on anecdotal evidence, however, as there has been no scientific research done on the subject. It is similar to the Binaca blast we talked about earlier in this book.

The Altoid urban legend was so pervasive, it was even featured in a "Sex Lessons" column from *Cosmopolitan* magazine a few years back. Of even more note, it is also mentioned in Kenneth Starr's report of the Clinton/Lewinsky sex scandal during Bill Clinton's term as President. After showing him the email, Monica slyly told the President she was chewing one at that very moment. For unknown reasons, President Clinton declined.

Question: Does fellatio prevent pre-eclampsia?

Pre-eclampsia is a condition in which a pregnant woman's blood pressure rises to potentially dangerous levels. The origin of the syndrome is not known. A recent entry in a European medical journal reported that women who performed fellatio on their partners before becoming pregnant had a significantly lower incidence of pre-eclampsia. However, one medical journal several years ago discovered that pre-eclamptic conditions decreased significantly in women whose obstetricians were able to make a solid emotional connection with them, thus pointing to possible psychological factors in pre-eclampsia. Could this be the case with the women and their partners? That fellatio merely created a stronger emotional bond? Or could it be, as surmised by the European journal, that the ejaculate was the preventative? The only way to know for sure is to know whether the women swallowed the ejaculate of their partners or not.

Question: Do you need a condom if you are a virgin?

"Virgin" is a term that is defined differently by different people, and it cannot be relied upon when determining your

Fellatio

sexual safety. While it may reduce your risk of picking up STDs, it does not completely eliminate the risks. There are some that can be transmitted in non-sexual ways. Some may be passed from mother to child during birth or may be picked up from things like sharing towels. For example, many people have oral herpes that they receive in total non-sexual ways, such as sharing drinks or a kiss from a relative. While condoms don't completely prevent the spread of oral herpes to the genitals of one's partner (or vise versa), they certainly do provide a great deal of protection. The best thing you can do when engaging in any sexual activity is to use barriers like condoms and dental dams in order to be safe.

Question: **Can an established couple ever consider foregoing the barriers during sexual activity?**

Both partners should have been monogamous for a least six months, with at least two clear STD screens. Each must show the other a printout of their test results. You should both be tested at least once a year from then on. Even with that six month period, there are still no guarantees.

Question: **Is it possible for a man to urinate during fellatio?**

It is extremely unlikely that any man is going to urinate into his partner's mouth by accident. Men cannot ejaculate and urinate at the same time. During ejaculation there is a reflex action that contracts a muscle in the neck of the bladder which leads to the penis preventing the flow of urine.

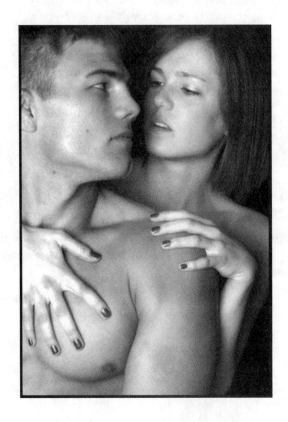

Figure 22: Men Have Emotional Needs too

15 The Emotional Needs of Men

Over-Simplification of Male Sexuality

Many years ago, there was a joke going around called "The Aggie Sex Manual." For the uninitiated, "Aggies" are people who attend or are alumni of Texas A&M University. The perception is that it is usually the naive country boy who attends this school (not true; just the perception). The manual consisted of three pages. Page one was an arrow pointing up which read "IN"; page 2 was an arrow pointing down which read "OUT"; page 3 read, "Repeat if Necessary." This is an eloquent illustration of the oversimplification of male sexuality. The common perception, which is often perpetuated in manuals and instruction books, is that all fellows want or need to do is stick it in, thrust once, and "repeat, if necessary." This is insulting to almost every man I know, who is much more than a penis. Unlike what many women say about men, they are not "led around by their penises." Nor is their every action dictated by the desires of their male member.

As a result of this kind of thinking and perpetuation of the myth, women believe that men are easy to please. This is often true, but we must think of our male partners as something more than machines that automatically respond without thought or feeling. He is capable of experiencing so much more than we give him credit for. It is our privilege and pleasure to see that he is fulfilled in every possible way. The gift of fellatio is for those who really care about the happiness and pleasure of their partners. It is not for amateurs who confine their men to one dimension.

Fellatio is meant to be enjoyed by both participants. Here is an excellent opportunity to be close to the one you love or desire. It is an erotic journey that is made more exciting because you are sharing it with each other. Your enjoyment will be mutual. Throw away your fears of doing something wrong. It is hard to do anything that is wrong when giving or receiving fellatio. The experience for the giver of your lips on his penis, and the experience for the receiver of the same, is unequaled. Do not worry if you are new to fellatio, or if you are merely trying a new position or technique. His gratitude and affection will be so great, it will only be surpassed by his patience in accepting your possibly clumsy ministrations. Relax, both of you, and the other party will respond accordingly. Enjoy the journey!

Index

Index

4

40-Year-Old Virgin, 46

6

69. *See* Sixty-Nine

A

Acupressure, 71, 72
African, 9
Art of Auto-Fellatio, 67
auto-fellatio, 1, 14, 67, 68

B

baboons, 11
Bill Clinton, 10, 114
Binaca Blast, 72
Bo Derek, 34
Bolero, 34

C

Caesar Milan, 20
Catholic Church, 9
chimpanzees, 11, 67
Cialis, 101
circumcision, 7, 31
cock and ball torture, 88
cockring, 7
condom, 45, 48, 93, 96, 97, 105, 106, 108, 109, 110, 111, 115
Condom(s), 110

D

Deep Throat, 10, 68
dildo, 49, 69, 70, 71, 91, 92
DNA, 64
Dog Whisperer, 20

E

Egypt, 8
ejaculate, 26, 27, 28, 35, 36, 37, 51, 63, 64, 75, 95, 102, 106, 114, 115
Ejaculate, 64
enema, 44
esophagus, 69

F

Family Business, 95
flogger, 89
Foreplay, 15
foreskin, 24, 27, 31, 44, 60, 109
frenulum, 24, 62

G

gagging, 58, 59, 69, 70

Gary Griffin, 67
gorilla
    moutain, 99
G-spot, 31, 62

H

Hepatitis, 105
HIV, 42, 105, 106
homosexual, 9, 14, 93
Hustler, 94

I

Impotency, 101
Inuit, 10
Iris, 8
Irrumation, 58
Islam, 9
Islamic. *See* Islam

J

Judeo-Christians, 9

K

Kama Sutra, 9

L

Levitra, 101
Linda Lovelace, 10, 68
lubricant, 80, 96, 97

M

massage
    erotic, 16
masturbation, 9, 29, 65, 66
Monica Lewinsky, 10
monogamous, 48, 107, 115

N

New Guinea, 9

O

Osiris, 8

P

penetration
    anal, 14
penis
    circumcised, 24
    implant, 84
    pierced, 53
    pump, 84
    size, 22
Penis
    enlargement, 84
plateau, 25, 27
Playboy, 94
Playgirl, 94
Pre-eclampsia, 114
pubic hair, 21, 44, 46

R

rimming, 61
Rimming, 61, 81, 97, 106
Rome, 9

S

S&M. *See* sadomachocism
sadomasochism, 85
scrotum, 24, 25, 32, 44, 46
sexually transmitted diseases, 10, 106
Seymour Butts, 95
Showtime, 95
Signature Solutions, 33
Silence of the Lambs, 47
Sixty-Nine, 82
STDs, 48
    sexually transmitted diseases, 106, 107, 115
strap-on, 3, 83, 91, 93

T

testicles, 21, 24, 27, 28, 44, 46, 57, 63, 80, 85, 88, 89, 90, 93
The Aggie Sex Manual, 117
The Silence of the Lambs, 47
transsexual, 14

U

University of Toronto, 22

Uprima, 101
urethra, 26, 28, 102

V

vibrators, 92

W

waxing, 46, 47
windpipe, 69

Glossary and Bibliography

Was that an earthquake?

Bibliography

The Sensuous Couple's Guide to Seismic Oral Sex

Bibliography

Videos

Hartley, Nina, *Making Love to Men*

Sinclair Institute, *Better Oral Sex Techniques*

Kramer, Joseph, *Fire on the Mountain: An Intimate Guide to Male Genital Massage*, 2007

Shopping

Austin (Forbidden Fruit)
Boston (Grand Opening)
New York (Toys in Babeland)
San Francisco (Good Vibrations)
Seattle (Toys in Babeland)
Toronto (Come as You Are, Good for Her)

Bibliography

Ryan, Vanessa, *The Master's Guide to Cunnilingus: How to Perform Successful Oral Sex and Provide the Highest Degree of Pleasure Possible*, Outskirts Press, Inc., outskirtspress.com, Denver, Colorado, Copyright 2006

Solot, Dorian and Miller, Marshall, *I Love Female Orgasm: An Extraordinary Orgasm Guide*, Marlowe and Company, Copyright 2007

Taylor, *You Want Me to Do What? An Illustrated Book on the Joys of Fellatio: Explicit Techniques*, Copyright 1999

Winks, Cathy and Semans, Anne, *The Good Vibrations Guide to Sex: The Most Complete Sex Manual Ever Written*, Cleis Press, Third Ed., Copyright 2002

Bibliography

Griffin, Gary M., *The Art of Auto-Fellatio (Oral Sex for One)*, Added Dimensions Publishing Inc., Raleigh, NC 27606, Fifth Edition, Copyright 2004

Heart, Mikaya, *When the Earth Moves; Women and Orgasm*, Celestialarts, Berkeley, California, Copyright 1998.

Hutchins, D. Claire, *Five Minutes to Orgasm Every Time You Make Love*, 2 Ed. by JPS Publishing Company, Midlothian, Texas, Copyright 2000

Joannides, Paul, *The Guide to Getting It On: A New and Mostly Wonderful Book About Sex for Adults of All Ages*, Group West Publishers, Berkeley, California, Copyright 2004 Goofy Foot Press

Kerner, Ian, Ph.D., *He Comes Next: The Thinking Woman's Guide to Pleasuring a Man*, HarperCollins Publishers, Inc., New York, NY, Copyright 2006

Kerner, Ian, Ph.D., *Passionista: The Empowered Woman's Guide to Pleasuring a Man*, HarperCollins Publishers, Inc., New York, NY, Copyright 2008

Kerner, Ian, Ph.D., *She Comes First: The Thinking Man's Guide to Pleasuring a Woman*, HarperCollins Publishers, Inc., New York, NY, Copyright 2004

Michaels, Marcy and Desalle, Marie, *The Low Down on Going Down: How to Give Her Mind-Blowing Oral Sex*, Broadway, Copyright 2004

Bibliography

Books

Allison, Dr. Sadie, *Tickle His Pickle*, 2004 2006©, Tickle Kitty, Inc., San Francisco, CA 94118

Birch, Robert W., *Oral Caress: The Loving Guide to Exciting a Woman: A Comprehensive Illustrated Manual on the Joyful Art of Cunnilingus*, PEC Publishing, Copyright 1996

Blue, Violet, *The Ultimate Guide to Cunnilingus: How to Go Down on a Woman and Give Her Exquisite Pleasure*, Cleis Press, Inc. San Francisco, California, Copyright 2002

Blue, Violet, *The Ultimate Guide to Fellatio: How to Go Down on a Man and Give Him Mind Blowing Pleasure*, Classic Press Inc., San Francisco, CA 94114, 1st Edition, Copyright 2002

Cage, Diana, *Box Lunch: The Layperson's Guide to Cunnilingus*, Alyson Books, Copyright 2004

Denchasy, Ian (Freddy) and Alicia (Eddy), *Art of Oral Sex: Bring Your Partner to New Heights of Pleasure*; Quiver, Copyright 2007

Fulbright, Yvonne K., *Touch Me There!: A Hands-On Guide to Your Orgasmic Hot Spots (Positively Sexual)*, Hunter House, Copyright 2007

Was that an earthquake?	The Sensuous Couple's Guide to Seismic Oral Sex
Bibliography	

Glossary

Vaginal farts — Occasionally air gets trapped in the vagina and makes fart like noise when it comes out. The action is normal and common and is most likely to happen upon orgasm when the rear part of the vagina which had ballooned open during arousal begins to collapse into its normal resting state.

Vanilla sex — Derogatory term refers to standard or conventional sex, usually the missionary position in heterosexual relationships. It can also refer to vaginal intercourse. Vanilla in English comes from the diminutive form of the Spanish word vaina, which means "scabbard" or "sheath" – the original meaning of the Latin word vagina.

Vestibular bulbs — Now thought by some to be part of the structure of the clitoris, these are filled with spongy tissue and swell with blood during arousal.

V-Spot — Slang term for frenulum.

Vulvio-vaginal candidiasis — A form of sexually transmitted disease, commonly known as yeast infection.

Yeast Infection — (See Vulvio-vaginal candidasis)

Glossary

STDs	Sexually transmitted diseases.	**Urethra**	The tube that brings semen and urine to the outside.
Syphillis	Bacterial infection transmitted primarily through sexual contact. Can be treated with antibiotics.	**Urethral opening**	Used for passing urine, is inside labia minor and lies between the introtus and the clitoral shaft and glans.
Taint	Nickname for perineum; i.e., "taint balls; taint butt."	**Uterus**	Pear shaped organ where a fetus can develop behind the vagina and between the bladder and rectum. The *uterus* is three inches long and two inches wide in a non-pregnant woman.
Tea bagging	A technique in which the balls of the man are sucked into the mouth of his partner.		
Terms	*Fellatio* comes from Latin term *fellare* which means "to suck." Use of the word "blowjob" in a sexual context was first recorded in 1961; as recently as 1953 it meant "type of airplane."	**Vagina**	Stretchable canal, about four inches long, that extends into the body and angles upward to the small of the back. It forms a flat tube when unaroused and expands much larger during childbirth. The walls of the vagina are moist and warm. When arousal occurs the walls are lubricated.
Testicles	Two round glands that produce sperm.		
Testosterone	A hormone that causes men to have beards, deep voices, muscles, sex drives and erections.		
Trichomonaisis	Bacterial form of sexually transmitted disease.		
Uncut	Refers to a penis that is uncircumcised.		

11

Glossary

Salmonella — A bacteria which causes food poisoning. The micro-organisms cause acute and vicious diarrhea and someone with mild symptoms may transmit the infection to someone else who develops severe symptoms.

Satyr — Generally human in appearance, but with a horse's tail and ears, the satyr was characterized by lust and cowardice, a symbol of the amoral and animalistic aspects of human nature.

Scrotum — The soft, wrinkled pouch that holds the testicles.

Shaft — The long neck of the penis from corona to scrotum.

Shigella — A bacteria which causes food poisoning. These micro-organisms cause acute and vicious diarrhea and someone with mild symptoms may transmit the infection to someone else who develops severe symptoms.

Sixty-Eight (68) — Oral sex position where the giver lies down, face up, with the receiver on top, also face up, in a head to toe fashion. The position is great for both cunnilingus and analingus.

Sixty-Nine (69) — Simultaneous reciprocal oral sex position in which both partners are mouth to genitals and perform oral sex on each other.

Smegma — The clitoral hood can accumulate *smegma*, a waxy substance, which can be prevented by pulling back the hood when washing.

Sphincters — Two circular muscles inside the anus designed to expand and contract.

Split Beaver — "Beaver" is slang for female genitals and split beaver is slang for when a woman holds her genitals open.

Squirting — The intense sexual arousal from the combination of oral sex, deep penetration and direct G spot stimulation may cause the female partner to "squirt," or ejaculate copiously.

Glossary

Perineum (female)	Smooth skin between anus and vaginal opening.
Pheromones	A sexually arousing chemical substance that is secreted into the air by many kinds of animals, including, possibly, humans.
Pre-come or pre-cum	A combination of fluid forced from the walls of the urethra and ejaculatory fluids processed in the prostatic urethra (where the fluids mix with semen before ejaculation).
Pre-eclampsia	A condition in which a pregnant woman's blood pressure can rise to potentially dangerous levels.
Pre-ejaculation	A slippery, clear or white liquid that oozes from the penis in varying amounts, long before orgasm, to provide lubrication.
Premature ejaculation (PE)	Also known as *rapid ejaculation, rapid climax, premature climax or early ejaculation*, is the most common sexual problem in men, affecting 25%-40% of men. It is characterized by a lack of voluntary control over ejaculation.
Prepuce	Foreskin.
Prostate	Muscular gland that creates fluid for semen.
Pubococ-cygeus muscle	The muscle that encircles the base of the penis and anus and pulses involuntarily at orgasm.
Rectum	Last segment of colon, or large intestine, the lowest part of the bowel found right before the anus.
Rimmer	Term for a person who engages in rimming.
Rimming	Slang term for *analingus*; the caressing or penetrating of one's lover's anal opening with the tongue.
Sack	Slang term for scrotum.
Sadism	The derivation of pleasure as a result of the suffering of others.
Sado-masochism	Sadism and masochism combined in one person.

Glossary

Oral sex — Consists of all sexual activities that involve the use of the mouth and tongue to stimulate genitalia. It may be used as foreplay before intercourse, as climax of a sexual act, or even following intercourse. It is sometimes performed to the exclusion of all other forms of sexual activity. Oral sex may or may not include the ingestion of semen and vaginal fluids. Ingestion of these fluids alone, without physical mouth-to genital contact (e.g., the extreme form of facial known as bukkake), is not considered to be oral sex. Common slang terms for oral sex include "going down on," "giving head to," "giving a blowjob to" (male), "eating out" (female), "licking out" (female) or sucking off" (male) a sexual partner.

Oral sex, cont. — Oral sex is often, but not always, intended to culminate in orgasm. Not only are the sexual organs sensitive and well supplied with nerve endings, the same is true of the mouth, tongue and lips, so enjoyment or oral sex is not always limited to the person on the receiving end.

Orgasm, one hour — The participants are said to enjoy high states of arousal for many hours and have a series of orgasms.

Os — Opening in cervix through which sperm and menstrual fluid can pass.

Ovaries — Female gonads that produce eggs and sex hormones.

Peehole — Slang term for the meatus.

Perineal sponge — Pad of spongy erectile tissue that lies between rectum and rear wall of vagina.

Perineum (male) — The nerve-ending-rich skin between the anus and the testicles.

Glossary

Hyman — Membrane of tissue covering introitus.

Interstitial cystitis — Interstitial cystitis (IC) is a condition that results in recurring discomfort or pain in the bladder and the surrounding pelvic region.

Introitus — Opening to the vagina.

Irrumation — Term for when the giver of fellatio stays stationary and the male receiving the fellatio provides the in and out motion with his thrusting.

Keefer — Slang expression for vaginal "farts." When air gets trapped in the vagina, it may make a fart-like noise when it comes out.

Labia majora — Outer lips of the vulva covered with pubic hair.

Labia minora — Inner lips around the vulva containing extensive blood vessels and nerve endings.

Masochism — A sexual perversion characterized by pleasure in being subjected to pain or humiliation especially by a love object.

Meatus — Refers to the two tiny lips at the tip of the penis head that are the tip of the urethra.

Monogamy — Relationship with only one other person.

Monosexuality — The complete avoidance of anyone other than one's self during any sex act.

Mons veneris — Female pubic mound.

Monsexual Movement — A movement advocating monosexuality.

Onanism — During the 19th century, any sexual act outside of coitus between a man and a woman was called by this name.

7

Glossary

Gokkun A Japanese semen fetish beyond the art of bukkake. Gokkun means literally "to gulp," which is the act of consuming large amounts of semen.

Gonorrhea Bacterial infection transmitted primarily through sexual contact. Can be treated with antibiotics.

Grafenburg spot Also known as the G spot, the area on the front wall of the vagina named for Ernest Grafenburg who described it in 1950. The *Grafenburg* spot is known as an area of erotic sensitivity when given manual stimulation.

Hepatitis Implies injury to the liver, a presence of inflammatory cells in the liver tissue. The condition can heal on its own or can progress to scarring of liver. It is called acute when it lasts less then 6 months and becomes chronic hepatitis when it persists longer. Hepatitis viruses cause most liver damage worldwide, but can also be due to toxins, particularly alcohol, other infections or from autoimmune process.

Hepatitis, cont. It may be asymptomatic at first but become symptomatic when the disease impairs liver functions that include among other things, screening of harmful substances, regulation of blood composition and production of bile to help digestion.

Hermaphrodite One having both male and female sexual characteristics and organs.

Herpes Herpes is an extremely contagious STD that is spread through contact with the mucous membranes of an infected person.

HIV The HIV virus is one of the causes of AIDS, a disease or cluster of diseases that involves a shutdown of the immune system.

HPV Human papillomavirus is the virus known as genital warts. It is transmitted through skin to skin and mucous membranes when the virus is shedding.

Hummer Slang term for fellatio.

Glossary

Fallopian tubes — The *fallopian tubes* are four inches long, extending from the uterus toward the ovaries. At the end of each tube are fringe-like projections called *fimbriae* that (after ovulation) draw the egg into the tube, where fertilization takes place.

Fellatio — Oral stimulation of the male genitals.

Fibroid tumors — Fibroid tumors are usually benign (non-cancerous) tumors found, most often, in the uterus of women in their 30's and 40's, although they occasionally develop on other organs. They are made of fibrous tissue, hence the name "fibroid" tumor. Most often fibroids occur as multiple tumor masses which are slow-growing and often cause no symptoms.

Fisting — Also known as *fist fucking*; a sexual activity that involves inserting the hand and forearm into the vagina or anus. This is not forcing the clenched fist; instead, all five fingers are kept straight and held as close together as possible (forming a beak-like shape, referred to as a "silent duck"), then slowly inserted into a well-lubricated vagina or anus. Once insertion is complete, the fingers either clench into a fist or remain straight. (from Wikepedia, the free encyclopedia: http://en.wikipedia.org/wiki/Fisting)

Fluid Bonded — When both partners have updated tests for STDs and infections and have agreed to have unprotected sex ONLY with each other.

Frenulum — The ultra-sensitive skin forming a "V" on the underside of the penis between the head and shaft.

Giving head — Slang term for fellatio.

Glans — Head or top part of penis designed for penetration.

Glossary

Double-dipping
Putting fingers, toys or anything else that has been in the anus to any other parts of the body, thereby transferring bacteria.

Ejaculation, Female
A gush of clear fluid from the urethral sponge.

Ejaculatory inevitability
The point-of-no-return at which a man's body gives him no choice but to ejaculate.

Embedded Clitoris
A clitoris which is completely hooded.

Endometriosis
Endometriosis is a common health problem in women. It gets its name from the word *endometrium*, the tissue that lines the uterus (womb). In women with this problem, tissue that looks and acts like the lining of the uterus grows outside of the uterus in other areas. These areas can be called growths, tumors, implants, lesions, or nodules.

Endometrium
Tissue that lines the interior wall of the uterus; the *perimetrium* is the thin outside covering and the smooth muscle layer of the wall is the *myometrium*.

Epiglottis
Thin structure behind the tongue that shields the entrance of the larynx during swallowing, preventing the aspiration of debris into the trachea and lungs.

Erotic Fantasy
Any thought, idea, image or scenario that is sexually arousing to an individual.

Facesitting
Also known as kinging or queening, involves sitting on or over the other partner's face, typically to allow oral-genital or oral-anal contact. It is common in dominance and submission, most common among dominant women and submissive men. The difference between facesitting and the similar practice of smothering is that smothering involves depriving the partner of air whereas facesitting does not.

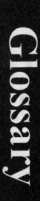

Glossary

Brazillian Wax — Waxing of the genital area where everything is waxed, including the anus, outer labia and inner labia.

Bukkake — Since directors could not show penetration, they had to invent new ways to approach sex acts that would satisfy the audience without violating the law. The act of drenching a woman in semen.

Bukkake, cont. — Popularized in Japan by adult video companies, a significant factor in its development was the mandatory censorship of porn in Japan. *Reverse bukkake* involves female ejaculation instead of male. The term "bukkake" was popularized in the United States by talk show host Howard Stern on his nationally syndicated radio program.

CBT — "Cock and ball torture" is administering erotic pain to the genitals, usually using toys or devices.

Cervix — End of the uterus in back of the vagina.

Chlamydia — Bacterial infection transmitted primarily through sexual contact. Can be treated with antibiotics.

Clitoris — Contains shaft and glans as well as crura, which projects inward from each side of the shaft; all contain spongy tissue called cavernous bodies. The clitoris swells during sexual arousal.

Clitoris, embedded — A completely hooded clitoris.

Corona — The tender ridge encircling the base of the penis head where it meets the shaft.

Cunnilingus — Act of using the mouth and tongue to stimulate the female genitals, especially the clitoris; comes from alternative Latin word for the vulva (*cunnus*) and from the Latin word for tongue (*lingua*).

Dental dam — Thick sheets of latex rubber that work like a condom, acting as a physical barrier between the anus and the mouth.

Glossary

Abstinence Programs Educational programs that teach that abstaining from sex is the only effective or acceptable method to prevent pregnancy or disease. They give no instruction on birth control or safe sex.

AIDS A disease or cluster of diseases that involve a shutdown of the immune system. The HIV virus is one of the causes of AIDS.

PC Muscles Pubococcygeal or PC muscle is the large sling of muscle that goes across the pelvic floor and supports the sexual organs. When tightened, the muscle can be felt in the clitoris, vagina, and anus.

Analingus Kissing, caressing or penetrating another's anal opening with the tongue. Anal oral contact, or analingus, is also known as rimming, rimjob, tossing the salad, pepe'ing, 87, or the black kiss. Analingus (from "anus" and "lingua," commonly misspelled as "analingus," compare to cunnilingus from "cunnus" and "lingua" is simultaneously anal sex and oral sex.

Anus Opening to the rectum.

Auto-Fellatio A practice whereby a man contorts himself into a position in which he is able to perform fellatio on himself.

Bacterial vaginosis (BV) Bacterial form of sexually transmitted disease.

Balls Slang term for testicles.

Beaver Slang for female genitals and split beaver is slang for when a woman holds genitals open.

Blowjob Slang term for fellatio.

GLOSSARY

Was that an earthquake? | The Sensuous Couple's Guide to Seismic Oral Sex